The Pilates Cadillac

Part II

The Leg Spring

Airplane Board

Arm Spring

Baby/Arm Chair Spring

Fuzzies and Cadillac Frame

Exercises

Reiner Grootenhuis

assisted by Dr. Ingo Barck

and Felicitas Ruthe

All photos of the Cadillac exercises: Photographer Miriam Abels; info@mimmoi.de
For all other photos see credits with the photo.
Cover photo: © I C Rapoport/icrapoport.com

All texts: Reiner Grootenhuis assisted by Dr. Ingo Barck and Felicitas Ruthe
Photo models: Helena Klimtova, Frank Staude, Claudia Holtmanns

Edited and translated by Talea Grootenhuis

ISBN: 9781697290776

Contact the author:

Reiner Grootenhuis

Email: info@pilates-powers.de

Telephone: +49 157 / 340 340 40

Website: http://www.pilates-powers.de

Table of Contents 1/4

Table of Contents 2/4

Table of Contents 3/4

Table of Contents 4/4

Preface Reiner Grootenhuis

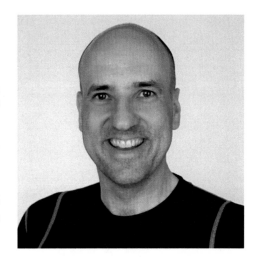

Working as a Pilates trainer is a great gift. Every hour is like a joint journey to the inner world. With its myofascial lines of traction and complex patterns of movement and compensation, the body constantly offers new discoveries and possibilities.

The Cadillac offers the most possibilities of all Pilates equipment to guide and shape such an inner journey. I try to convey the joy of discovering it together in this second part.

In the first part of the Cadillac Manual, published in English in April 2019, we began the manual with an introduction to the Cadillac, including a list of all the components of the Cadillac, the history of the Cadillac, and a comparison of classic and modern variants. We also presented the basic risks of working with springs, highlighted the Cadillac-specific safety risks and gave tips on how to use the manual.

The main part obviously consisted of the over 100 exercises with the Roll-Down-Bar and the Push-Through-Bar.

Since the release of the first part, the manual has been very well received by the Pilates community and is now Amazon's best-rated Cadillac manual if you sum up the reviews from Amazon.com and Amazon.de.

In this second part of the Cadillac Manual, we continue with the Leg Springs, Airplane Board, Arm Springs and Baby/Arm Chair Springs exercises, as well as the work with the Cadillac frame and the Fuzzies exercises.

We purposely decided not to repeat the introductory part and instead begin directly with the exercises.

I wish you a lot of fun with using this manual and trying out all the exercises and would be very happy to receive your questions and feedback.

Tönisvorst (Germany), October 2019   Reiner Grootenhuis

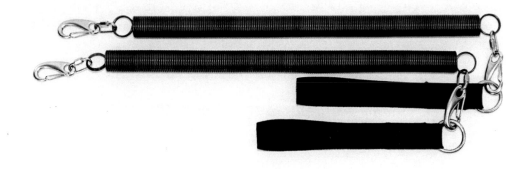

Leg Springs

Preliminary Remarks for the Leg Springs

The repertoire of exercises with the feet in the "Leg Springs" on the Cadillac is considerably wider than that of comparable Reformer exercises. Another special feature of working with the leg springs compared to working with the loops on the Reformer is that the on the Reformer, the straps are always connected to the carriage via the pulley at the back end of the Reformer and, therefore, both legs always experience the same resistance. If one leg now presses harder than the other, this will not be visible from the outside. It becomes more visible on the Cadillac as the legs work with independent springs. The same considerations later apply to the arm work with the arm springs as opposed to the arm work on the Reformer.

How an exercise with the leg springs works depends strongly on the springs being used. The philosophy of the springs varies from manufacturer to manufacturer, whereby the biggest difference can be seen between the springs of Deborah Lessen and those of other manufacturers. Deborah Lessen has her springs produced in the tradition of her teacher Carola Trier. The peculiarity is that her springs offer an increased resistance at the beginning and a more even resistance when stretched. With other manufacturers, the beginning is usually rather soft and the further the spring is stretched, the stronger the spring force becomes. As it happens so often, it is not possible to say which of the two philosophies is the right one. In our Pilates Studio we use springs from different manufacturers, including those from Deborah Lessen.

Traditionally, the heavy leg springs on the Cadillac are attached at a height of 83.5 cm / 32.8 inches. Meanwhile, the attachment on Carola Trier's Cadillac was at 31.5 inches, which is equivalent to 80 cm. Since we know that Carola Trier's equipment was built by Joseph Pilates at least at the beginning, it is reasonable to assume that he had lowered the leg springs for Carola Trier due to her smaller body size. Joseph Pilates used a similar procedure for the Reformer, which he built for the smaller Eve Gentry, by making the Reformer slightly smaller in size.

In addition to the more traditional springs, the use of long soft leg springs has also become popular, which are then attached much higher. Since there is a danger of slipping out of these loops, the use of Y-loops or loops like the ones being used in Gyrotonic® is advisable.

Although, as described in the first part of the manual, there was no predetermined order, certain series have been established for this work, though it is difficult to say whether they came from Joseph Pilates himself. The series for the leg springs is:

- Leg Circles (Cadillac-wide)

- Walking 8 Counts

- Beats

- Bicycle

- Little Circles

1. Frog (T)
1/2

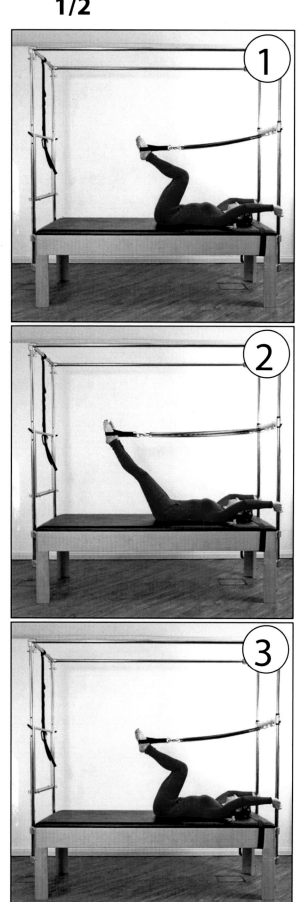

1. Frog (T)
2/2

Setup:

Attach traditional leg springs at a height of 80 - 85 cm / 31.5 - 33.5 inches. The higher the spring attachment, the more the leg backsides have to work.

Supine position with the head pointing toward the spring attachments. The distance to the vertical bars of the Cadillac should be between half an arm-length and one arm-length. The further away, the harder the exercise. The hands hold the vertical bars slightly above the shoulders. Pelvis in a neutral position, spine in a natural position. Feet in the loops, the loops are in the arch of the foot, tendentially closer to the heels. The legs are slightly rotated outward and bent. <u>Feet in a small V</u> (heels together, toes apart) and stretched. The feet are slightly above the knees. The knees are shoulder-wide apart. Frog position.

Purpose of the Exercise:

Mobilization of the hip.
Using the ischiocural musculature as movement initiators.
Strengthening of the hip and knee extensors.
Strengthening of the ankles and foot extensors.
Decoupling the leg movement from the hip and torso.

Execution: 5x - 10x

Pull the abdomen inward and upward. Stabilize the entire trunk with the muscles.
Stretch the legs simultaneously and completely.
The stability of the pelvis and lower back is maintained.
Bend the legs while resisting the springs, returning to the starting position.

Common Mistakes:

The pelvis tilts with the movement of the legs.
The knees are too far apart in the starting position.
The legs rotate inward while straightening.
The contact between the heels is given up and the heels move into opposite directions.

Modifications or Variations:

Move your feet back and forth at exactly the same height when stretching and bending your legs.
For very tall people, the use of a loop with a longer loop or the use of an additional carabiner can lengthen the leg springs so that the force at the end of the movement is not too great.
Change of pace after the first five repetitions. First 5 slowly, then 5 faster.
Attach long, soft leg springs at a higher point on the Cadillac, if possible with Y-loops or gyro-double-loops that run both along the arch and around the ankle of the foot.

Contraindications/Risks:

The exercise should be omitted with traditional leg springs in case of the following pre-existing conditions: acute herniated discs, osteoporosis.

2. Big Circular Frog (T)

1/3 Alternative name: Big Frog, Frog in 6 counts

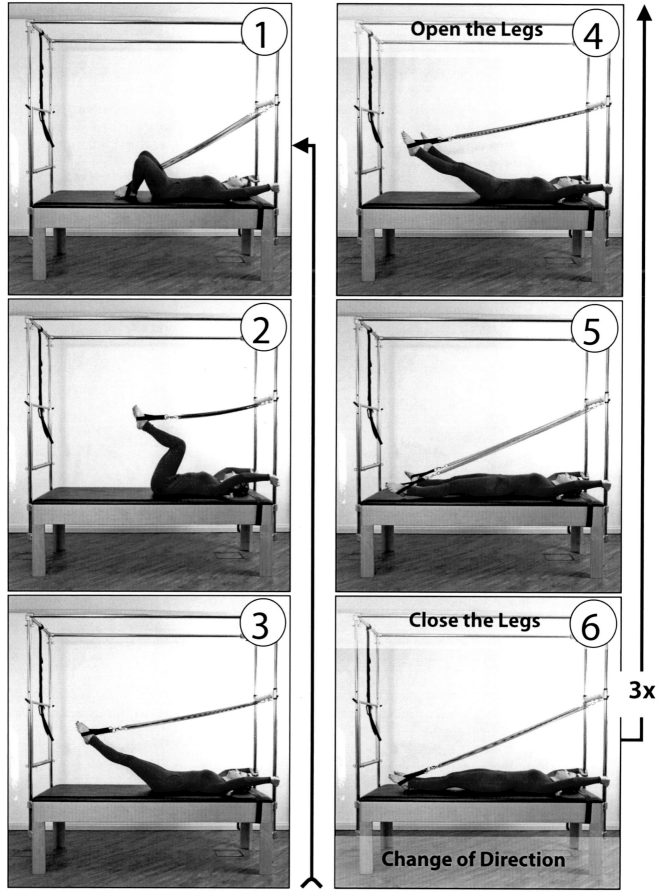

1

2

3

4 — Open the Legs

5

6 — Close the Legs

Change of Direction

3x

2. Big Circular Frog (T)

2/3 Alternative name: Big Frog, Frog in 6 counts

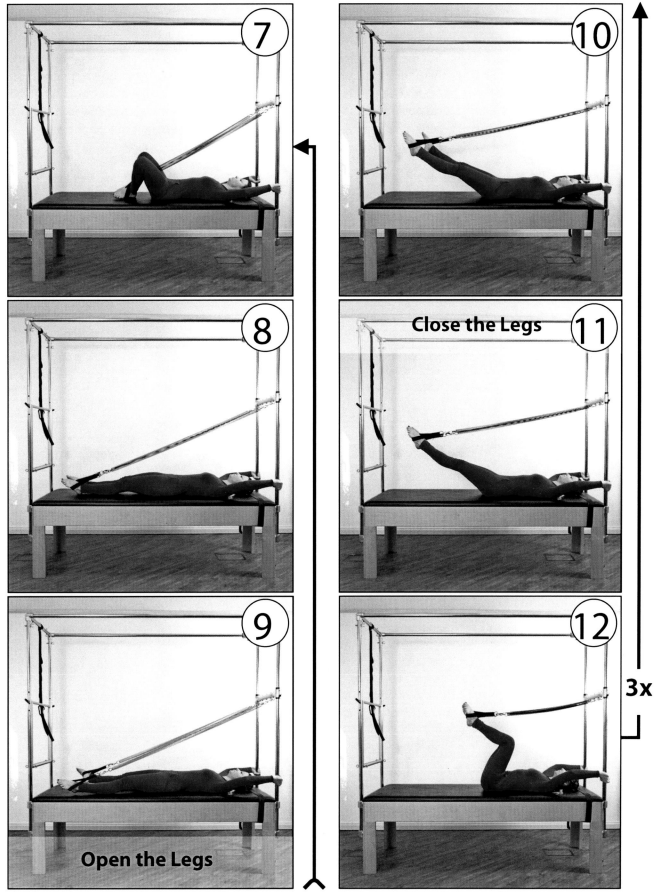

2. Big Circular Frog (T)

3/3 Alternative name: Big Frog, Frog in 6 counts

Setup:

Attach traditional leg springs at a height of 80 - 85 cm / 31.5 - 33.5 inches. The higher the spring attachment, the more the leg backsides have to work. Supine position with the head pointing toward the spring attachments. The distance to the vertical bars of the Cadillac should be between half an arm-length and one arm-length. The further away, the harder the exercise. The hands hold the vertical bars slightly above the shoulders. Pelvis in a neutral position, spine in a natural position. Feet in the loops, the loops are in the arch of the foot, tendentially closer to the heels. The legs are slightly rotated outward and bent. <u>Feet in a small V</u> (heels together, toes apart) on the mat behind the buttocks. The knees are shoulder-wide apart.

Purpose of the Exercise:

Mobilization of the hip.
Strengthening of the hip and knee extensors.
Decoupling the leg movement from the hip and torso.
Coordinative training. Training the movement memory.

Execution: 3x -5x per side

Pull the abdomen inward and upward. Stabilize the entire trunk with the muscles.

Image 2:   (1) Bring the legs into the frog position.
Image 3:   (2) Stretch the legs simultaneously and completely.
Image 4:   (3) Open the legs as wide as the Cadillac, keeping them at the same height.
Image 5:   (4) Evenly lower the legs onto the Cadillac mat. The legs remain stretched.
Image 6:   (5) Bring the slightly outward rotated legs together on the Cadillac surface. Feet in a small V.
Image 1:   (6) Bend the legs and pull the feet across the Cadillac mat and toward the buttocks. The knees are shoulder-wide apart. The springs are between the legs.

Repeat 3x - 5x, then change the direction.

Image 7:   The legs are slightly rotated outward and bent. Feet in a small V on the mat behind the buttocks. The knees are shoulder-wide apart. The springs are between the legs.
Image 8:   (1) Stretch the legs simultaneously and completely.
Image 9:   (2) Open the legs Cadillac-wide, leaving them on the Cadillac mat.
Image 10:   (3) Raise the legs to approx. 45 degrees, keeping them at them Cadillac-wide apart.
Image 11:   (4) Close the legs, keeping them at 45 degrees. The legs remain stretched.
Image 12:   (5) Bend the legs and come back into the frog position. The knees are shoulder-wide apart.
Image 7:   (6) Put the legs down on the Cadillac mat, the feet standing close to the buttocks. Feet in a small V.

Common Mistakes:

The stability of the pelvis is neglected.
The height of the feet varies with the movement forward and backward, instead of remaining steady.
Loss of concentration and confusion of the movement sequence.

Modifications or Variations:

For very tall people, the use of a loop with a longer loop or the use of an additional carabiner can lengthen the leg springs so that the force at the end of the movement is not too great.
Attach long, soft leg springs at a higher point on the Cadillac, if possible with Y-loops or gyro-double-loops that run both along the arch and around the ankle of the foot.

Contraindications/Risks:

The exercise should be omitted with traditional leg springs in case of the following pre-existing conditions:

3. Dolphin & Dolphin Reverse (M)
1/3

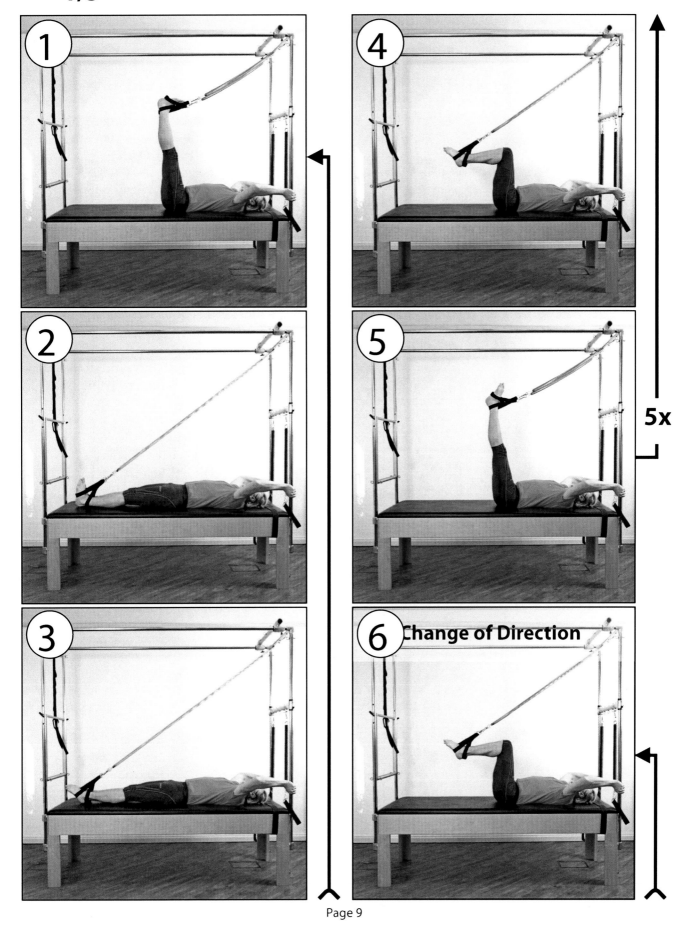

3. Dolphin & Dolphin Reverse (M)
2/3

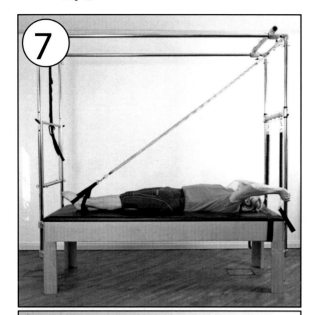

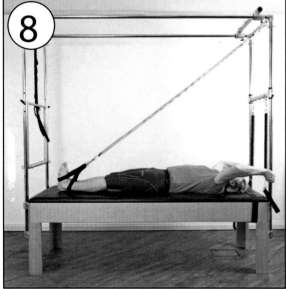

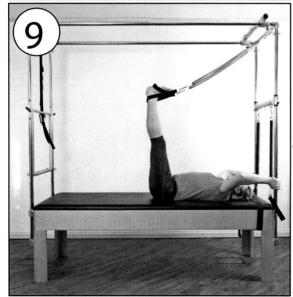

5x

Setup:

Select the spring position so that the exercise can be performed completely and without any evasive movements. The height of the spring position also influences the effect of the exercise. Typically, the long, soft leg springs are attached at the highest possible point of the Cadillac. Ideally, use Y-loops or gyro-double-loops that run both along the arch and around the ankle of the foot.

Supine position with the head pointing toward the spring attachments. The distance to the vertical bars of the Cadillac should be between half an arm-length and one arm-length. The further away, the harder the exercise. The springs should not hang loosely when the legs are vertical. The hands hold the vertical bars slightly above the shoulders or lie alongside the body. Pelvis in a neutral position, spine in a natural position. The feet are in the loops. The legs are parallel, closed with inner tension and stretched out vertically. If the vertical position cannot be reached while maintaining a natural spinal position (danger of a posterior pelvic tilt and pressure on the lumbar spine), move the legs upward only as long as the hip remains stable. The feet are parallel and flexed. Soles of the feet are on one level from the heels, over the outer side of the foot, the ball of the foot to the toes. The toes are slightly opened and relaxed.

Purpose of the Exercise:

Mobilization of the hip.
Decoupling the leg movement from the hip and torso.
Strengthening of the hip and knee extensors and the leg adductors.
Stretch of the leg backsides.
Coordinative training.
Training the movement memory.

3. Dolphin & Dolphin Reverse (M)
3/3

Execution: 5x - 10x per side

Pull the abdomen inward and upward. Stabilize the entire trunk with the muscles.

Image 2:   Bring the legs downward onto the Cadillac mat with stretched feet.

Image 3:   Stretch the feet, the toes closing and maintain the leg position.

Image 4:   Bring the legs into the tabletop position. Make sure to move the shins parallel to the Cadillac mat on the way there. Avoid excessively bending the knees. Picture of a tray with champagne glasses, which you do not want to tip over. Therefore, the springs also do not touch the legs.

Image 5:   Stretch the legs up vertically - the feet remain stretched on the way up. The knees remain in the same spot and are not pulled toward the body. 90 degree angle of the legs to the pelvis. After the stretch, flex the feet and open the toes.

Repeat 5x - 10x, then change the direction.

Image 6:   From the position with upward stretched legs, stretch the feet up and bend the legs back into tabletop position. The knees remain in the same spot and are not pulled toward the body.

Image 7:   Lower the stretched legs. Make sure to move the shins parallel to the Cadillac mat on the way there. Avoid excessively bending the knees. Picture again a tray with champagne glasses, which you do not want to tip over.

Image 8:   Flex the feet, open the toes slightly - maintain the lower leg position.

Image 9:   Move the stretched legs upward. Maintain the flexion of the feet throughout the movement.

Repeat 5x - 10x.

Common Mistakes:

The stability of the pelvis is neglected.

The feet sickle (supination) in the extension and the flexion.

The inner thigh tension is given up and the legs move slightly independently from each other.

The legs are raised further than 90 degrees, or the thighs are pulled toward the body when bending.

The springs go beyond neutral spring tension and make a clicking noise.

Modifications or Variations:

Perform the exercise "over the frame", see exercise "10. Bicycle over the Frame". Alternatively, you can do the exercise on two Reformer boxes. This allows the legs to be moved below the Cadillac support surface or the surface of the Reformer boxes. Take care not to fall into the hollow back.

Contraindications/Risks: -

4. Walking (T)
1/3

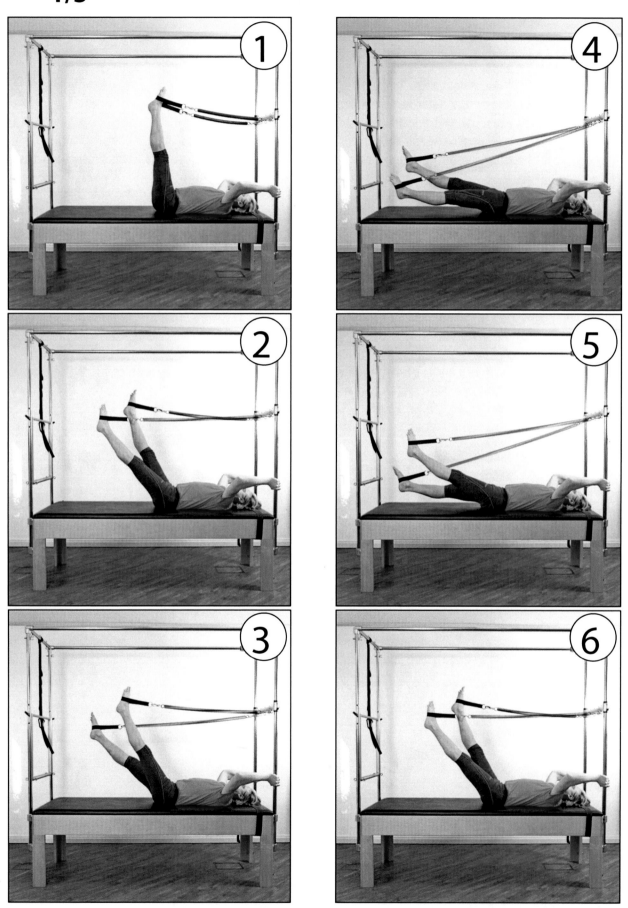

4. Walking (T)
2/3

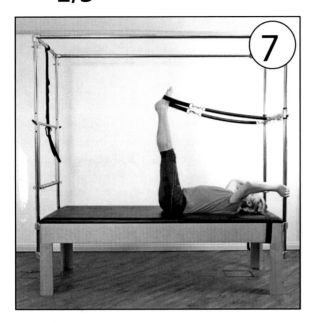

Setup:
Attach traditional leg springs at a height of 80 - 85 cm / 31.5 - 33.5 inches. The higher the spring attachment, the more the leg backsides have to work.
Supine position with the head pointing toward the spring attachments. The distance to the vertical bars of the Cadillac should be between half an arm-length and one arm-length. The further away, the harder the exercise. The hands hold the vertical bars slightly above the shoulders. Pelvis in a neutral position, spine in a natural position. Feet in the loops, the loops are in the arch of the foot, tendentially closer to the heels. <u>The legs are parallel</u> and stretched upward. <u>Feet stretched.</u>

Purpose of the Exercise:
Mobilization of the hip and the sacroiliac joint.
Strengthening of the hip and knee extensors.
Decoupling the leg movement from the hip and torso.
Coordinative training.

Execution: 3x - 7x
Pull the abdomen inward and upward. Stabilize the entire trunk with the muscles.
Image 2-4: Walk downward in 8 quick steps, keeping the legs stretched. The step size is relatively small. If possible, touch the Cadillac mat softly with the last step.
Image 5-7: Walk upward in 8 quick steps, keeping the legs stretched. The step size remains relatively small.

Common Mistakes:
The stability of the pelvis is neglected.
The feet sickle (supination) in the extension.
The inner thigh tension is given up.
The legs are raised further than 90 degrees.
The springs go beyond neutral spring tension and make a clicking noise.

4. Walking (T)
3/3

Modifications or Variations:

For very tall people, the use of a loop with a longer loop or the use of an additional carabiner can lengthen the leg springs so that the force at the end of the movement is not too great.

If a vertical position of the legs cannot be reached while maintaining a natural spinal position (danger of a posterior pelvic tilt and pressure on the lumbar spine), slide toward the spring attachments and/or lengthen the springs through carabiners or longer loops. The legs are thereby lowered. In addition in case, be careful not to raise the legs completely vertically.

Attach long, soft leg springs (approx. 31 inches / 79 cm length) at a higher point on the Cadillac, if possible with Y-loops or gyro-double-loops that run both along the arch and around the ankle of the foot.

Perform the exercise "over the frame", see exercise "10. Bicycle over the Frame".

Contraindications/Risks: -

5. Beats (T)
1/2

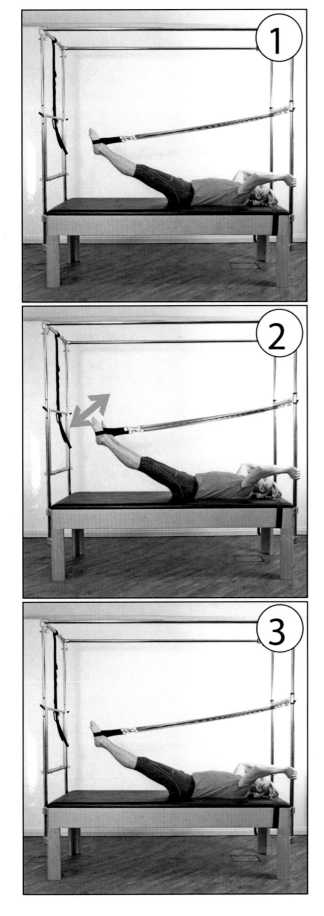

5. Beats (T)
2/2

Setup:
Attach traditional leg springs at a height of 80 - 85 cm / 31.5 - 33.5 inches. The higher the spring attachment, the more the leg backsides have to work.

Supine position with the head pointing toward the spring attachments. The distance to the vertical bars of the Cadillac should be between half an arm-length and one arm-length. The further away, the harder the exercise. The hands hold the vertical bars slightly above the shoulders. Pelvis in a neutral position, spine in a natural position. Feet in the loops, the loops are in the arch of the foot, tendentially closer to the heels. Legs stretched to approx. 45 degrees. The legs are in a slight outward rotation, <u>feet in a small V</u> (heels together, toes apart) and stretched.

Purpose of the Exercise:
Strengthening of the inner thighs.
Coordinative training.
Maintaining control over the springs.

Execution: 3 sets with up to 10 repetitions
Pull the abdomen inward and upward. Stabilize the entire trunk with the muscles.
Separate the heels slightly and then close them, initiated from the leg adductors, dynamically and quickly. Perform the entire exercise on one level.
10 repetitions. Pause.
10 repetitions. Pause.
10 repetitions.

Common Mistakes:
The springs begin to vibrate in one of their own natural frequencies, which can build up. Instead, keep the springs as steady as possible and counteract the proper motion of the springs.
The heels are knocked together too strongly. Instead, emphasize the initiation from the inner thighs.

Modifications or Variations:
Perform the three sets at three different heights.
If the heels are pounded too hard, alternatively emphasize the movement outwards instead of inwards.
For very tall people, the use of a loop with a longer loop or the use of an additional carabiner can lengthen the leg springs so that the force at the end of the movement is not too great.
Attach long, soft leg springs (approx. 31 inches / 79 cm length) at a higher point on the Cadillac, if possible with Y-loops or gyro-double-loops that run both along the arch and around the ankle of the foot.

Contraindications/Risks: -

6. Small Leg Circles (T)
1/3

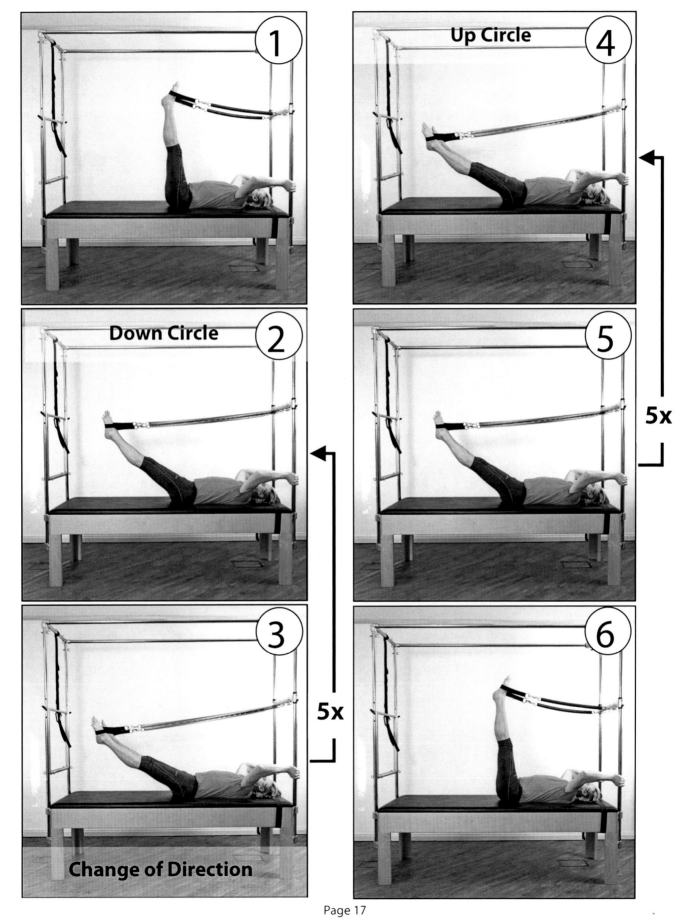

6. Small Leg Circles (T)
2/3

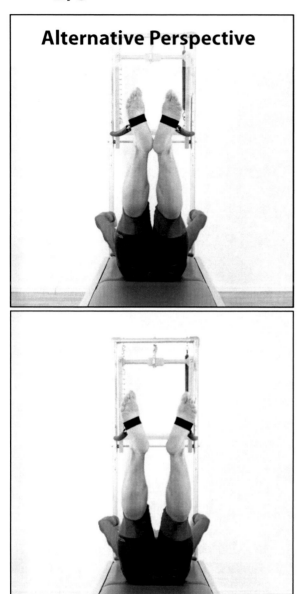

Alternative Perspective

6. Small Leg Circles (T)
3/3

Setup:
Attach traditional leg springs at a height of 80 - 85 cm / 31.5 - 33.5 inches. The higher the spring attachment, the more the leg backsides have to work.

Supine position with the head pointing toward the spring attachments. The distance to the vertical bars of the Cadillac should be between half an arm-length and one arm-length. The further away, the harder the exercise. The hands hold the vertical bars slightly above the shoulders. Pelvis in a neutral position, spine in a natural position. Feet in the loops, the loops are in the arch of the foot, tendentially closer to the heels. The legs are stretched upward. The legs are in a slight outward rotation, <u>feet in a small V</u> (heels together, toes apart) and stretched.

Purpose of the Exercise:
Strengthening of the entire leg musculature and hip extensors within a small radius of motion.
Coordinative training.

Execution: 5x 10x
Pull the abdomen inward and upward. Stabilize the entire trunk with the muscles.
Lower the closed legs to approx. 45 degrees.

Down Circle
Lower the closed legs to approx. 30 - 40 degrees.
Open the legs about foot-wide (max. foot-long).
Raise the legs in a semicircle to approx. 45 degrees and close them.

5-10 repetitions, then change the direction.

Up Circle
Open the legs about foot-wide (max. foot-long) at approx. 45 degrees.
Lower the legs in a semicircle to approx. 30 - 40 degrees and close them.
Lift legs closed again to approx. 45 degrees.

5-10 repetitions, then bring the legs back to their vertical position.

Common Mistakes:
Lack of precision in the execution.
The circle is too wide.
The small V is given up.
Lack of pelvic stability.

Modifications or Variations:
For very tall people, the use of an additional carabiner can lengthen the leg springs so that the force at the end of the movement is not too great.
Attach long, soft leg springs at a higher point on the Cadillac, if possible with Y-loops or gyro-double-loops that run both along the arch and around the ankle of the foot.

Contraindications/Risks: -

7. Leg Circles (T)
1/3

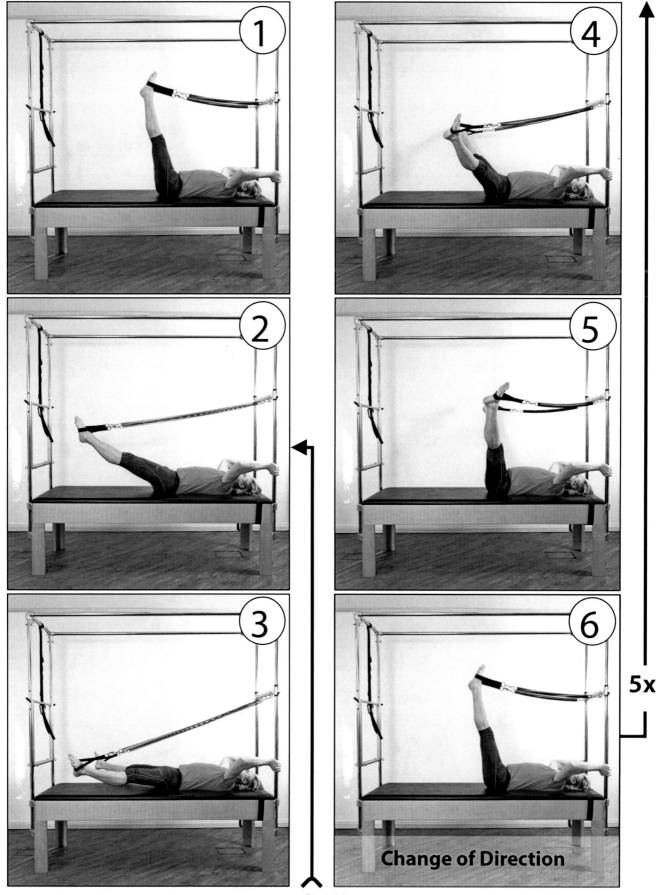

Change of Direction

5x

7. Circles (T)
2/3

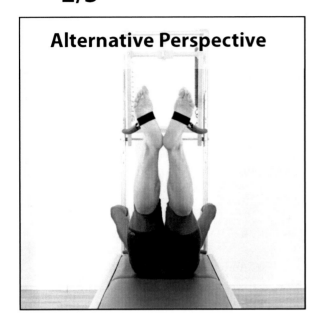

Alternative Perspective

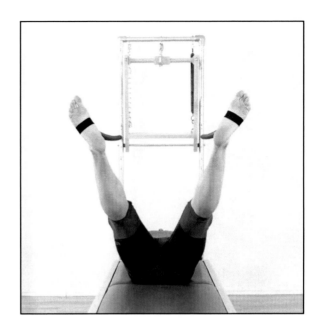

Setup:

Attach traditional leg springs at a height of 80 - 85 cm / 31.5 - 33.5 inches. The higher the spring attachment, the more the leg backsides have to work.

Supine position with the head pointing toward the spring attachments. The distance to the vertical bars of the Cadillac should be between half an arm-length and one arm-length. The further away, the harder the exercise. The hands hold the vertical bars slightly above the shoulders. Pelvis in a neutral position, spine in a natural position. Feet in the loops, the loops are in the arch of the foot, tendentially closer to the heels. The legs are stretched upward.

The legs are in a slight outward rotation, <u>feet in a small V</u> (heels together, toes apart) and stretched.

Purpose of the Exercise:

Strengthening of the entire leg musculature, especially the adductors and hip extensors.
Mobilization of the hips.

Execution: 5x -10x

Pull the abdomen inward and upward. Stabilize the entire trunk with the muscles.

Down Circle

Keeping the legs closed as much as possible, lower them without otherwise changing the body position. Then open the legs and move them to the sides, raising them in a large "D" and finally closing them again. 5-10 repetitions, then change the direction.

Up Circle

Move the legs to the sides from the vertical leg position and lower them in a large "D". Finally, close them again and bring them upward, still stretched and in a small V.
5-10 repetitions, then change the direction.

7. Circles (T)
3/3

Common Mistakes:

The mobility of one leg to the outside is greater, resulting in the side with the restriction pulling the pelvis to its restricted side. Make the circles smaller accordingly.

The springs are released more quickly in the upward direction than in the downward. The speed should remain constant.

The springs are completely released by tilting the pelvis upward so that they suddenly hang through. Do not raise the springs this high.

Modifications or Variations:

For very tall people, the use of an additional carabiner can lengthen the leg springs so that the force at the end of the movement is not too great.

If a vertical position of the legs cannot be reached while maintaining a natural spinal position (danger of a posterior pelvic tilt and pressure on the lumbar spine), slide toward the spring attachments and/or lengthen the springs through carabiners. The legs are thereby lowered. In addition or alternatively, be careful not to raise the legs completely vertically.

Attach long, soft leg springs at a higher point on the Cadillac, if possible with Y-loops or gyro-double-loops that run both along the arch and around the ankle of the foot.

Perform the exercise "over the frame", see exercise "10. Bicycle over the Frame".

Instead of a precise "D" shape, for the " Down Circles", alternatively do not press the legs down all the way to the mat, and when moving the legs to the side, come a little lower and only then back up. At the top, too, first come down a little before the legs are brought together. The movement reminds of two full circles with a slightly longer line in the center. As a reference picture the magnetic field of a rod magnet can be used. Compared to the standard version with the "D", less adductor work is necessary here. However, this version is more dynamic and has more work in the abductors and outer rotators of the legs.

Move the feet in two rectangles instead of circles.

In the "D", maintain parallel legs instead of the small V.

A more extensive flex and point variation, best using softer springs from above:
Start with the Up Circle
The legs are parallel, closed and vertical, the feet are flexed. Particularly make sure to pull the outer edge of the small toe toward the knee. Rotate the legs as far outward as possible. Then, move the legs outward, and, using the entire radius of motion, downward. At about half way, stretch the feet. Continue the movement and finally close the legs. The legs are parallel. Flex the feet and move the legs upward, tightly closed.
5-10 repetitions, then continue *with the Down Circle*
With the legs in a vertical position, stretch the feet and lower them as far as possible. Then, flex the feet, rotate the legs outward and raise them in a large "D". There, close the legs parallely and stretch the feet again.
5-10 repetitions, then change the direction.

Contraindications/Risks:

Danger of luxation in case of fresh hip endoprostheses.

8. Scissors (T)
1/2

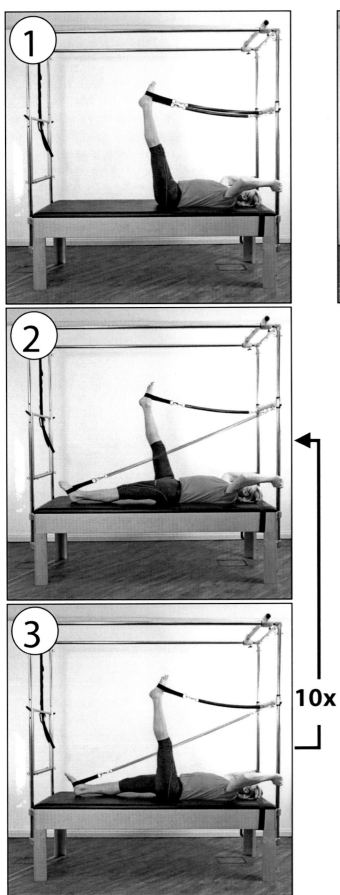

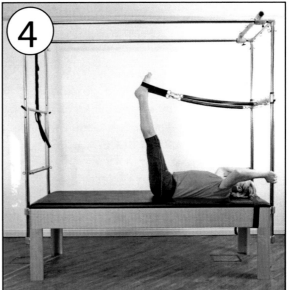

10x

8. Scissors (T)
2/2

Setup:

Attach traditional leg springs at a height of 80 - 85 cm / 31.5 - 33.5 inches. The higher the spring attachment, the more the leg backsides have to work.

Supine position with the head pointing toward the spring attachments. The distance to the vertical bars of the Cadillac should be between half an arm-length and one arm-length. The further away, the harder the exercise. The hands hold the vertical bars slightly above the shoulders. Pelvis in a neutral position, spine in a natural position. The feet are in the loops, the loops are in the arch of the foot, tendentially closer to the heels. The legs are parallel and stretched upward. Feet stretched. If a vertical position of the legs cannot be reached while maintaining a natural spinal position (danger of a posterior pelvic tilt and pressure on the lumbar spine), slide toward the spring attachments and/or lengthen the springs through carabiners. The legs are thereby lowered. In addition or alternatively, be careful not to raise the legs completely vertically.

Purpose of the Exercise:

Strengthening of the knee extensors, leg backsides and hip extensors.
Mobilization of the hip and the sacroiliac joint.

Execution: 10x

Pull the abdomen inward and upward. Stabilize the entire trunk with the muscles.
Move one leg as far downward as possible without otherwise changing the body position. While the leg is moving back up, the other leg is moved downward. Viewed from the side, there is a large "L" at the end positions with one leg at the top and one at the bottom. During the exercise, always make sure in in both directions - up and down - to reach the maximum length of the leg and foot without moving the pelvis along. The idea is to constantly extend the leg away from the hip. Particularly during the upward movement, make sure to extend the thigh as far away from the hip as possible.

Common Mistakes:

The pelvis constantly tilts along with the leg movement.
The mobility of one leg is more extensive and the movement is therefore not performed evenly.
The speed of the legs in the upward movement is faster than in the downward movement, which goes against the spring resistance.
One leg is raised so high that the spring hangs through. Increase the distance to the spring attachments or raise the springs less high up.

Modifications or Variations:

To enhance the feeling of extending the thigh bone away from the hip in the upward movement, use the side of the hand to push the raising leg away directly at the base of the leg.
For very tall people, the use of an additional carabiner can lengthen the leg springs so that the force at the end of the movement is not too great.
Attach long, soft leg springs at a higher point on the Cadillac, if possible with Y-loops or gyro-double-loops that run both along the arch and around the ankle of the foot.
Perform the exercise in a small V with a slight outward rotation of the legs.
Perform the exercise in an maximum outward rotation.
Perform the exercise "over the frame", see exercise "10. Bicycle over the Frame".
Instead of stretching both feet, flex both feet.
Flex the feet in the upward movement. Stretch the feet in the downward movement. And the other way around: point upward, flex downward.

Contraindications/Risks: -

9. Bicycle (T)
1/4

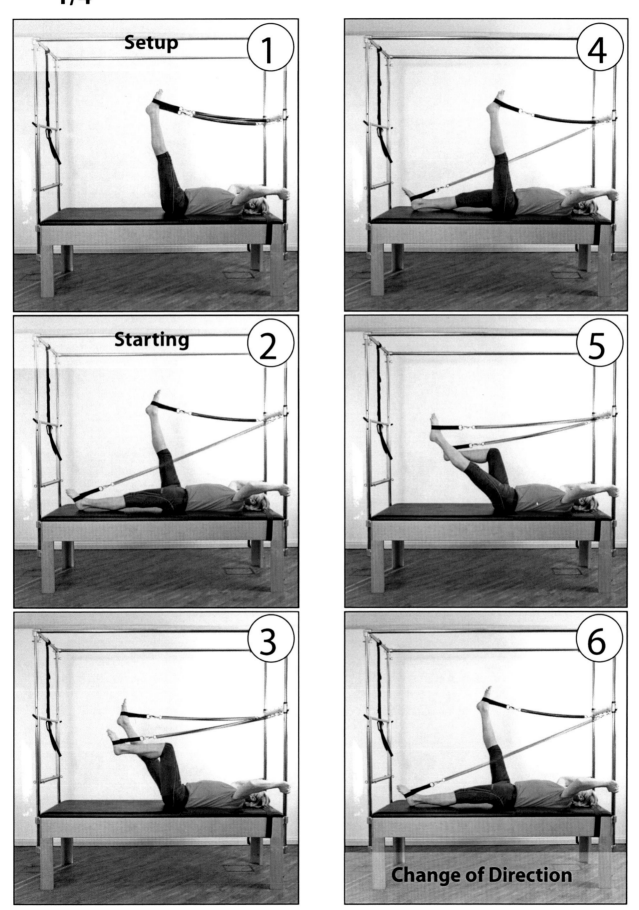

9. Bicycle (T)
2/4

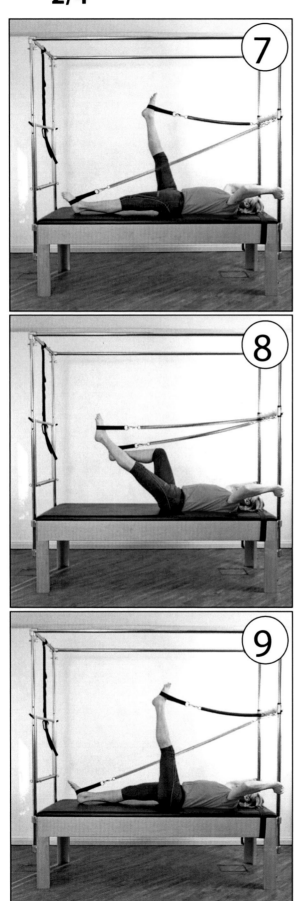

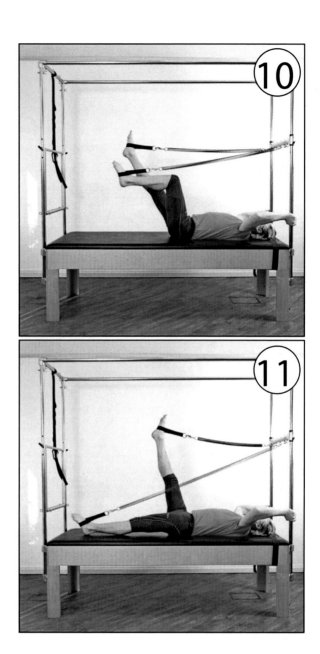

9. Bicycle (T)
3/4

Setup:

Attach traditional leg springs at a height of 80 - 85 cm / 31.5 - 33.5 inches. The higher the spring attachment, the more the leg backsides have to work.

Note: Even though the Bicycle exercise is a traditional exercise, as an exception, an alternative way of execution is shown first. For the traditional exercise, please use the description under "Modifications or Variations".

Supine position with the head pointing toward the spring attachments. The distance to the vertical bars of the Cadillac should be between half an arm-length and one arm-length. The further away, the harder the exercise. The hands hold the vertical bars slightly above the shoulders. Pelvis in a neutral position, spine in a natural position. The feet are in the loops, the loops are in the arch of the foot, tendentially closer to the heels. <u>The legs are parallel</u> and stretched upward. <u>Feet stretched.</u>

If a vertical position of the legs cannot be reached while maintaining a natural spinal position (danger of a posterior pelvic tilt and pressure on the lumbar spine), slide toward the spring attachments and/or lengthen the springs through carabiners. The legs are thereby lowered. In addition or alternatively, be careful not to raise the legs completely vertically.

Purpose of the Exercise:

Strengthening of the knee extensors, knee flexors and hip extensors.
Mobilization of the hip and the sacroiliac joint.
Improvement of the coordinative abilities.

Execution: 5x - 10x per direction

Pull the abdomen inward and upward. Stabilize the entire trunk with the muscles.

Image 2: Lower the stretched left leg.

Image 3: As the left leg is bent, the right leg already begins the way down. While bending the left leg, make sure that the shin is always parallel to the Cadillac mat. Imagine balancing a plate on the shin until it reaches the tabletop position. The spring never touches the shin.

Image 4: As soon as the left knee is exactly above the hip (tabletop position), stretch the leg out upward. Keep the knee right above the hip and do not pull it any further. The right leg is now completely laid down on the mat.

Image 5: Move the left leg down stretched while the right leg is already on its way upward. While bending the right leg, make sure that the shin is always parallel to the Cadillac mat.

Image 6: As soon as the right knee is exactly above the hip (tabletop position), stretch the leg out upward. Keep the knee right above the hip and do not pull it any further. The left leg is now completely laid down on the mat.

Repeat 5x-10x, then change the direction.

Common Mistakes:

The pelvis constantly tilts along with the leg movement.
One leg is raised so high that the spring hangs through. Increase the distance to the spring attachments.
While bending, the knee is pulled further, so the thigh surpasses 90 degrees.

9. Bicycle (T)
4/4

Modifications or Variations:

In the traditional version of the exercise, the legs are rotated outward with the knees pointing outward and the springs running on the inside.

Perform the exercise with only one leg to get more accuracy into the sequence of movements. The unused leg can either lie on the mat without a spring, stand on the mat, or hang in the spring stretched out but passively.

Attach long, soft leg springs at a higher point on the Cadillac, if possible with Y-loops or gyro-double-loops that run both along the arch and around the ankle of the foot.

Perform the exercise "over the frame", see exercise "10. Bicycle over the Frame".

Instead of stretching both feet, flex both feet.

Flex the foot in the upward movement. Stretch the foot in the downward movement. And the other way around: point upward, flex downward.

Contraindications/Risks: -

10. Bicycle over the Frame (M)
1/4

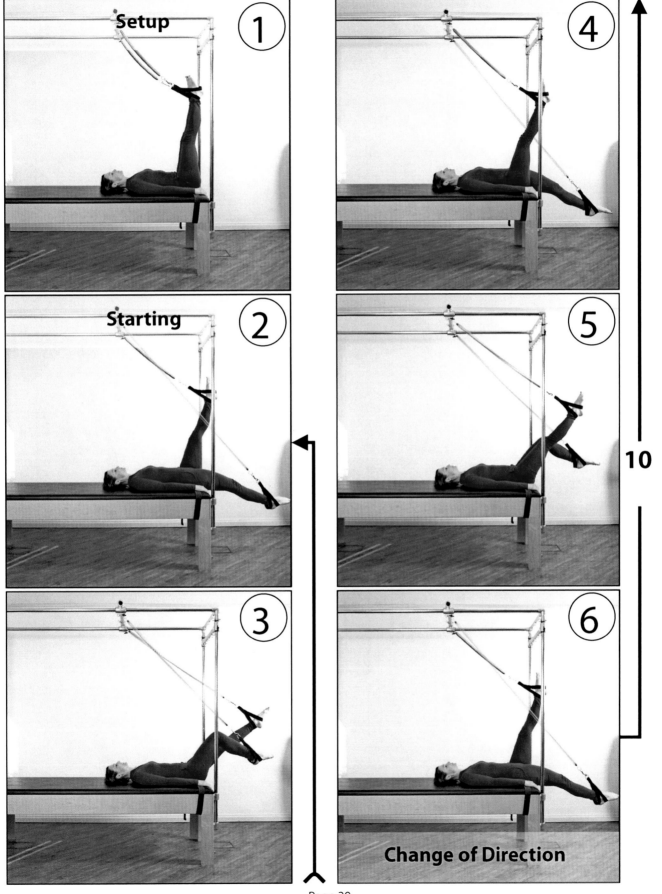

10. Bicycle over the Frame (M)
2/4

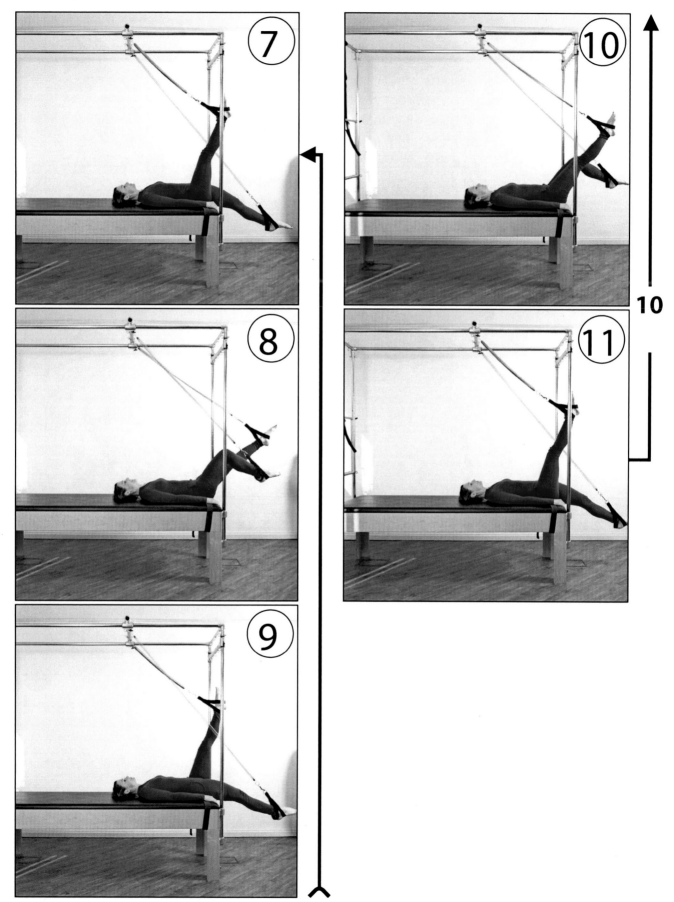

10. Bicycle over the Frame (M)
3/4

Setup:

Attach long leg springs to the attachment of the Trapeze Bar. The attachment is positioned above the face.
Supine position with the head looking up at the spring attachments, pointing into the Cadillac. Pelvis in a neutral position, spine in a natural position. Feet in the loops, if possible with Y-loops or gyro-double-loops that run both along the arch and around the ankle of the foot. <u>The legs are parallel</u> and stretched upward. <u>Feet stretched.</u> If a vertical position of the legs cannot be reached while maintaining a natural spinal position (danger of a posterior pelvic tilt and pressure on the lumbar spine), slide toward the spring attachments and/or lengthen the springs through carabiners. The legs are thereby lowered. In addition or alternatively, be careful not to raise the legs completely vertically.

Purpose of the Exercise:

Strengthening of the knee extensors, leg backsides and hip extensors.
Stretching of the deep hip flexors.
Mobilization of the hip and the sacroiliac joint.
Improvement of the coordinative abilities.

Execution: 5x - 10x per direction

Pull the abdomen inward and upward. Stabilize the entire trunk with the muscles.

Image 2:	Lower the right stretched leg as far down as possible. Do not pull the lower back into a hollow position and avoid a winging of the ribs.
Image 3:	As the right leg is bent, the left leg already begins the way down. While bending the right leg, make sure that the shin is always parallel to the Cadillac mat. The leg holds the tension.
Image 4:	As soon as the right knee is exactly above the hip (tabletop position), stretch the leg out upward. Keep the knee right above the hip and do not pull it any further. The left leg has already reached its lowest position at this point.
Image 5:	Move the right leg down stretched while the left leg is already on its way upward. While bending the left leg, make sure that the shin is always parallel to the Cadillac mat.
Image 6:	As soon as the left knee is exactly above the hip (tabletop position), fully stretch the leg upward. Keep the knee right above the hip and do not pull it any further. The right leg has already reached its lowest possible position at this point.

Repeat 5x-10x, then change the direction.

Common Mistakes:

The pelvis constantly tilts along with the leg movement.
The lower back is pulled into a hollow position.
The leg is not lowered as far as possible and the other leg is not fully stretched upward.
One leg is raised so high that the spring hangs through. Adjust the position of the Trapeze Bar attachment.

10. Bicycle over the Frame (M)
4/4

Modifications or Variations:

Legs in maximum outer rotation, feet in Charlie Chaplin position.

Perform the exercise with only one leg to get more accuracy into the sequence of movements. The unused leg can either lie on the mat without a spring, stand on the mat, or hang in the spring stretched out but passively.

Instead of stretching both feet, flex both feet.

Flex the foot in the upward movement. Stretch the foot in the downward movement. And the other way around: point upward, flex downward.

On the Tower/Wall Unit, the position can also be replicated by using two vertical Reformer Boxes and a correspondingly high attachment of the leg springs. Alternatively, a limited extension of the legs can also be reached by using a MoonBox, a ball or a Pilates roll below the pelvis.

Contraindications/Risks:

Danger of luxation in case of fresh hip endoprostheses. Hence, do not move downward via the horizontal position and instead better perform exercise "9. Bicycle".

11. Lower Legs Lift (M)
1/2

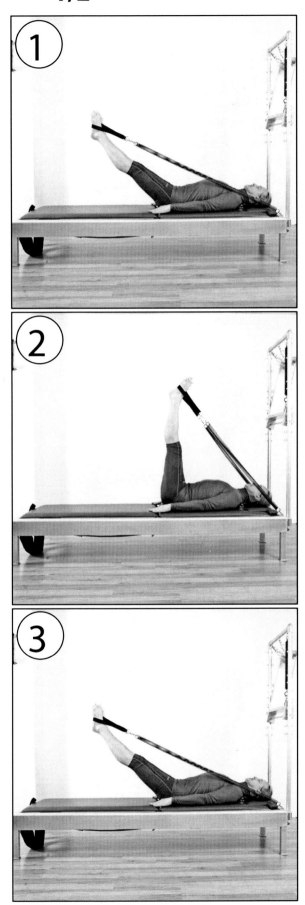

11. Lower Legs Lift (M)
2/2

Setup:

If possible, attach traditional leg springs at mat height. Supine position with the head pointing toward the spring attachments. The distance to the vertical bars of the Cadillac should be between half an arm-length and one arm-length. The further away, the harder the exercise. Place the outstretched arms on the mat, lying closely alongside the body. Slight pressure across the entire back of the arm and pressure of the hands into the mat. Pelvis in a neutral position, spine in a natural position. Feet in the loops, the loops are in the arch of the foot, tendentially closer to the heels. The legs are in a slight outward rotation, <u>feet in a small V</u> (heels together, toes apart) and stretched. Bring the legs to approx. 45 degrees so that the springs are just above the shoulders, not coming into contact with them.

Purpose of the Exercise:

Stabilization of the pelvis.
Strengthening of the knee extensors, leg backsides and hip extensors.

Execution: 5x - 7x

Pull the abdomen inward and upward. Stabilize the entire trunk with the muscles.
Move the legs together and closed as far up into a vertical position as possible without changing the pelvic position. This also means that the lumbar spine does not move during the exercise.
Lower the legs into the starting position again.

Common Mistakes:

The pelvis tilts up with the movement and the lumbar spine is flattened.

Modifications or Variations:

For very tall people, the use of an additional carabiner can lengthen the leg springs so that the force at the end of the movement is not too great.
To make the exercise more demanding, slide a little further away from the spring attachments. This also allows for a deeper angle of the legs to be chosen.
Use traditional leg springs at a height of 80 - 85 cm/31.5 - 33.5 inches.
To make the movement of the lumbar spine visible to customers, the Chattanooga STABILIZER™ Pressure Bio-Feedback has proven to be useful. Place the STABILIZER™ cuff beneath the lumbar spine and inflate the chambers to 40 mmHg/approx. 40,000 millitorr (the abbreviation for millimeter of mercury - derived from analog blood pressure monitors). Perform the "Lower Leg Lift" exercise, keeping the value of 40 mmHg/40.000 millitorr as constant as possible. Alternatively, an analogue blood pressure monitor, which is often cheaper to obtain, can also be used as feedback. However, the two supply lines from the manometer to the upper arm cuff are then usually made of a softer material and if you lie down on it, e.g. with the pelvic edge, the line is interrupted and the value on the manometer is no longer reliable.

Contraindications/Risks: -

12. Reformer based Frog (M)

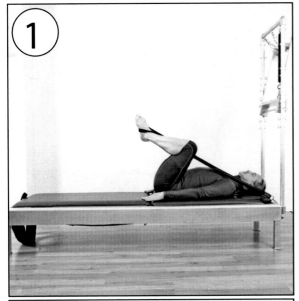

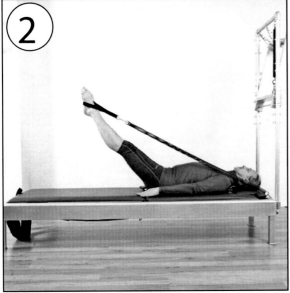

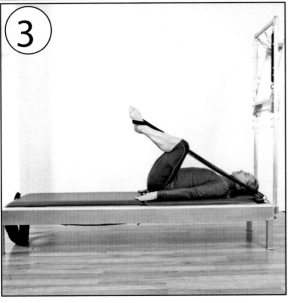

Setup:

If possible, attach traditional leg springs at mat height. Supine position with the head pointing toward the spring attachments. The distance to the vertical bars of the Cadillac should be between half an arm-length and one arm-length. The further away, the harder the exercise. Place the outstretched arms on the mat, lying closely alongside the body. Slight pressure across the entire back of the arm and of the hands into the mat. Pelvis in a neutral position, spine in a natural position. Feet in the loops, the loops are in the arch of the foot, tendentially closer to the heels. The legs are in a slight outward rotation, <u>feet in a small V</u> (heels together, toes apart) and stretched. Bend the legs with the knees shoulder-wide apart. The feet are slightly above the knees. Frog position.

Purpose of the Exercise:

Stabilization of the pelvis.
Strengthening of the knee extensors and inner thighs.

Execution: 5x - 10x

Pull the abdomen inward and upward. Stabilize the entire trunk with the muscles.
Stretch the legs upward to approx. 45 degrees, the springs run just above the shoulders, not coming into contact with them. Initiate the stretch from the inner thighs. Shortly keep the legs stretched before bending them again.

Common Mistakes:

The knees are wider than the shoulders, meaning that there is a lack of inner thigh tension at the beginning. The movement is performed too much by the knee extensors.
The legs are stretched upward almost vertically.

Modifications or Variations:

For very tall people, the use of an additional carabiner can lengthen the leg springs so that the force at the end of the movement is not too great.
To make the exercise more demanding, slide a little further away from the spring attachments. This also allows for a deeper angle of the legs to be chosen.

Contraindications/Risks: -

13. Reformer based Openings (M)
1/2

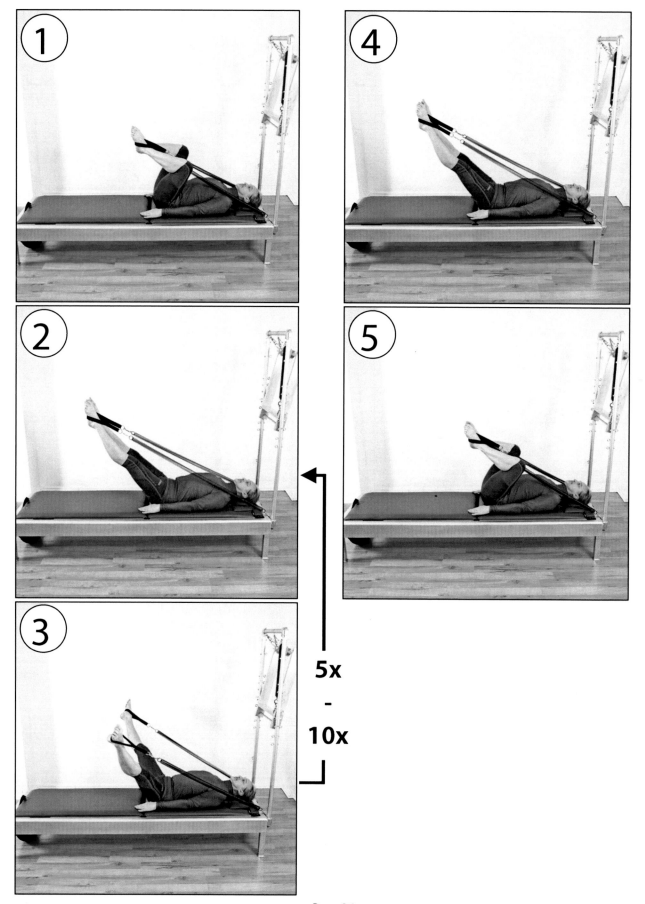

5x
-
10x

13. Reformer based Openings (M)
2/2

Setup:
If possible, attach traditional leg springs at mat height. Supine position with the head pointing toward the spring attachments. The distance to the vertical bars of the Cadillac should be between half an arm-length and one arm-length. The further away, the harder the exercise. Place the outstretched arms on the mat, lying closely alongside the body. Slight pressure across the entire back of the arm and of the hands into the mat. Pelvis in a neutral position, spine in a natural position. Feet in the loops, the loops are in the arch of the foot, tendentially closer to the heels. The legs are in a slight outward rotation, <u>feet in a small V</u> (heels together, toes apart) and stretched. Bend the legs with the knees shoulder-wide apart. The feet are slightly above the knees. Frog position.

Purpose of the Exercise:
Stabilization of the pelvis.
Strengthening and stretch of the inner thighs.

Execution: 5x - 10x
Pull the abdomen inward and upward. Stabilize the entire trunk with the muscles.
Stretch the legs upward to approx. 45 degrees, the springs run just above the shoulders, not coming into contact with them. Initiate the stretch from the inner thighs. Shortly keep the legs stretched.
Then move the legs outward until a comfortable stretch of the inner thighs is achieved.
After 5x-10 x repetitions, return the legs to the starting position.

Common Mistakes:
On the way back to the starting position, the legs are moved upward from the stretch almost vertically and from there to the sides instead of moving them into the position at approx. 45 degrees.

Modifications or Variations:
For very tall people, the use of an additional carabiner can lengthen the leg springs so that the force at the end of the movement is not too great.
To make the exercise more demanding, slide a little further away from the spring attachments. This also allows for a deeper angle of the legs to be chosen.
To stretch other parts of the adductors, bring the legs to 90 degrees and from there open them to the sides. Use traditional leg springs at a height of 80 - 85 cm/31.5 - 33.5 inches instead.

Contraindications/Risks:
In case of sensitive knees, make sure that the movement is not continued to the very end of the radius of motion and is thereby "decoupled". If the feeling at the end of the outward movement is uncomfortable, bend the knees for safety reasons and only then bring them back together.

14. Reformer based Extended Frog (M)
1/3

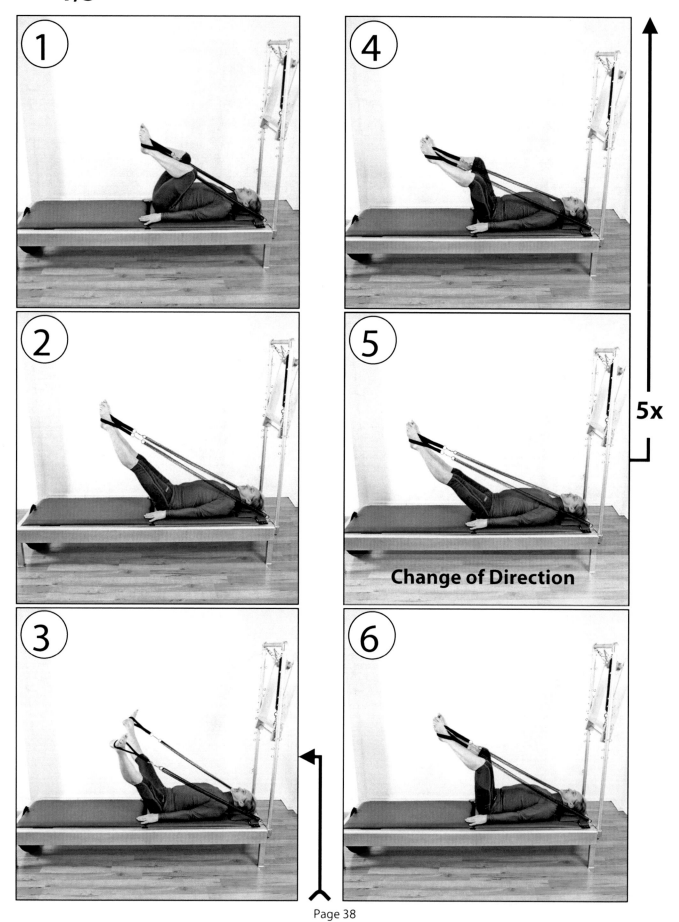

14. Reformer based Extended Frog (M)
2/3

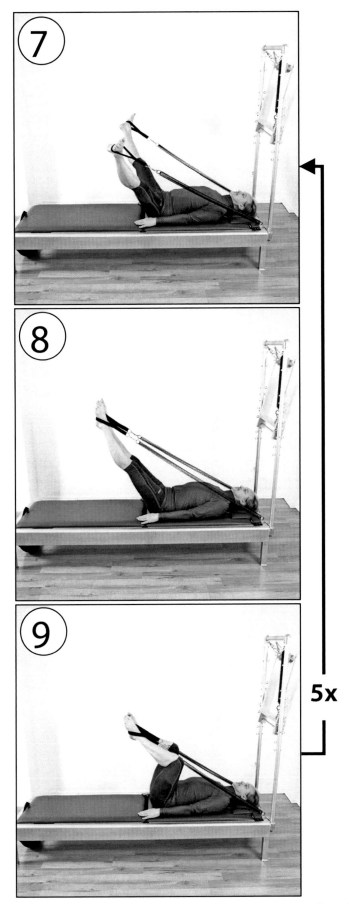

5x

14. Reformer based Extended Frog (M)
3/3

Setup:
If possible, attach traditional leg springs at mat height. Supine position with the head pointing toward the spring attachments. The distance to the vertical bars of the Cadillac should be between half an arm-length and one arm-length. The further away, the harder the exercise. Place the outstretched arms on the mat, lying closely alongside the body. Slight pressure across the entire back of the arm and of the hands into the mat. Pelvis in a neutral position, spine in a natural position. Feet in the loops, the loops are in the arch of the foot, tendentially closer to the heels. The legs are in a slight outward rotation, <u>feet in a small V</u> (heels together, toes apart) and stretched. Bend the legs with the knees shoulder-wide apart. The feet are slightly above the knees. Frog position.

Purpose of the Exercise:
Stabilization of the pelvis.
Strengthening of the leg backsides and knee extensors.
Strengthening and stretch of the inner thighs.

Execution: 5x - 7x per direction
Pull the abdomen inward and upward. Stabilize the entire trunk with the muscles.
Image 2-5: Stretch the legs upward to approx. 45 degrees, the springs run just above the shoulders, not coming into contact with them. Initiate the stretch from the inner thighs. Shortly keep the legs stretched. Then move the legs outward until a comfortable stretch of the inner thighs is achieved.
Bend the legs and close the heels again. As far as possible, move only the lower legs in the knee joint. The thighs are not moved, it feels like the knees pull to the sides. The legs form a diamond shape. Imagine reaching around a large ball with the legs.
Then stretch the legs again. After 5x - 7x repetitions change the direction.
Image 6-9: The legs are in the diamond or slightly more bent like in the frog position. Open the legs and, as far as possible, move only the lower legs in the knee joint. The thighs are not moved. Close the legs, the feet remaining at the same height. Bend the legs again. Repeat 5x - 7x.

Common Mistakes:
While closing the heels, the position of the thighs is given up. Same problem after the change of direction when opening the thighs.

Modifications or Variations:
For very tall people, the use of an additional carabiner can lengthen the leg springs so that the force at the end of the movement is not too great.
To make the exercise more demanding, slide a little further away from the spring attachments. This also allows for a deeper angle of the legs to be chosen.
Use traditional leg springs at a height of 80 - 85 cm/31.5 - 33.5 inches.
Attach long, soft leg springs at a higher point on the Cadillac, if possible with Y-loops or gyro-double-loops that run both along the arch and around the ankle of the foot.
Instead of performing the exercise at approx. 45 degrees, it can also be performed with soft leg springs (attached at a higher position), with traditional leg springs (attached at 80 - 85 cm/31.5 - 33.5 inches), on the Cadillac mat or as close as possible and parallel to the Cadillac mat.

Contraindications/Risks: -

15. Reformer based Short Spine (M)
1/3

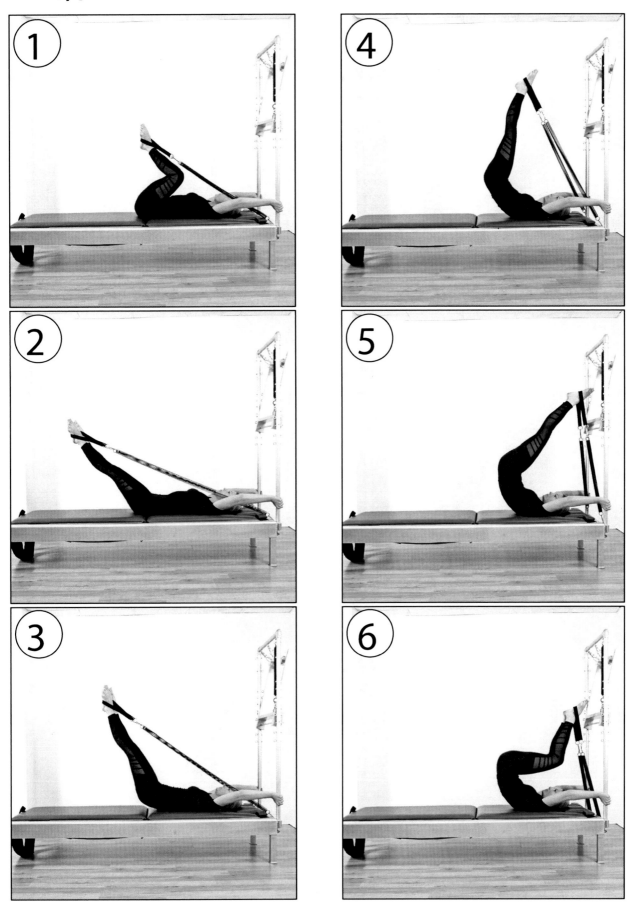

15. Reformer based Short Spine (M)
2/3

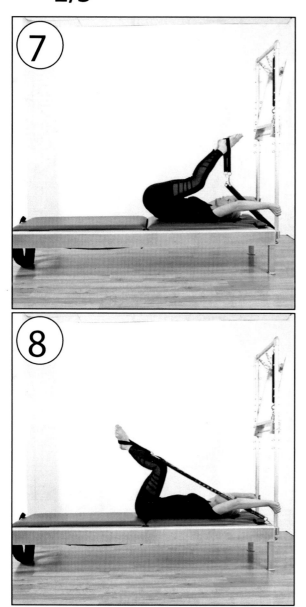

15. Reformer based Short Spine (M)
3/3

Setup:
If possible, attach traditional leg springs at mat height. Supine position with the head pointing toward the spring attachments. The distance to the vertical bars of the Cadillac should be between half an arm-length and one arm-length. The hands hold the vertical bars slightly above the shoulders. Pelvis in a neutral position, spine in a natural position. Feet in the loops, the loops are in the arch of the foot, tendentially closer to the heels. The legs are in a slight outward rotation, <u>feet in a small V</u> (heels together, toes apart) and stretched. Bend the legs with the knees shoulder-wide apart. The feet are slightly above the knees. Frog position.

Purpose of the Exercise:
Mobilization and stretch of the entire spine with focus on the lumbar spine.
Stretch of the leg backsides through the extension of the legs in the diamond position.

Execution: 3x - 7x
Image 2: Stretch the legs upward to approx. 45 degrees, the springs run just above the shoulders, not coming into contact with them. Initiate the stretch from the inner thighs. Shortly keep the legs stretched.
Image 3: Tilt the pelvis posteriorly and slightly raise it, using the abdominal muscles. The legs only move toward the spring attachments as far as necessary.
Image 4-5: While maintaining the angle between the torso and the legs, bring the feet above the head. Make sure to go only as far as not to exert any pressure on the cervical spine. Ideally, in this position the head can just barely still be lifted.
Image 6: Let the feet stay above the head, the hips holding the height, and bend the knees about shoulder-wide.
Image 7: With the feet still above the head, roll the back down slowly. The knees widen outward and make room for the chest. The legs form a diamond.
The two movements in images 6 and 7 are harder on the Cadillac than on the Reformer as the springs are relaxed at this point, requiring the arms, shoulders and abdominals to keep the weight of the body from rolling down.
Image 8: Roll down the rest of the back. At the same time, pull the feet toward the buttocks. Roll down until a neutral pelvic position is reached and the legs are back in the starting position.

Common Mistakes:
In images 2-5 the legs are brought backward too much by the springs. The body is "folded" with the head flat on the knees. Instead, take an active position, rounded with some space between the head and knees like an inverted Teaser, so the lower back can be extended. No stretch!
In images 6-7 the movement becomes imprecise and too fast due to the lack of spring support.
In images 4-6, too much pressure is exerted on the cervical spine.

Modifications or Variations:
Instead of opening the knees when rolling down, keep the knees closed.
Instead of working without tensioning of the springs when rolling down, after the 90/90 position (picture 6), the rolling of the spine is combined with a forward tilting of the legs, so that the springs are constantly under light tension.
The High Frog from the Reformer can also be done here.

Contraindications/Risks:
The exercise causes an increased strain on the shoulder and should therefore only be performed by people with healthy shoulders.
In the overhead positions, make sure that the cervical spine is not overstrained.

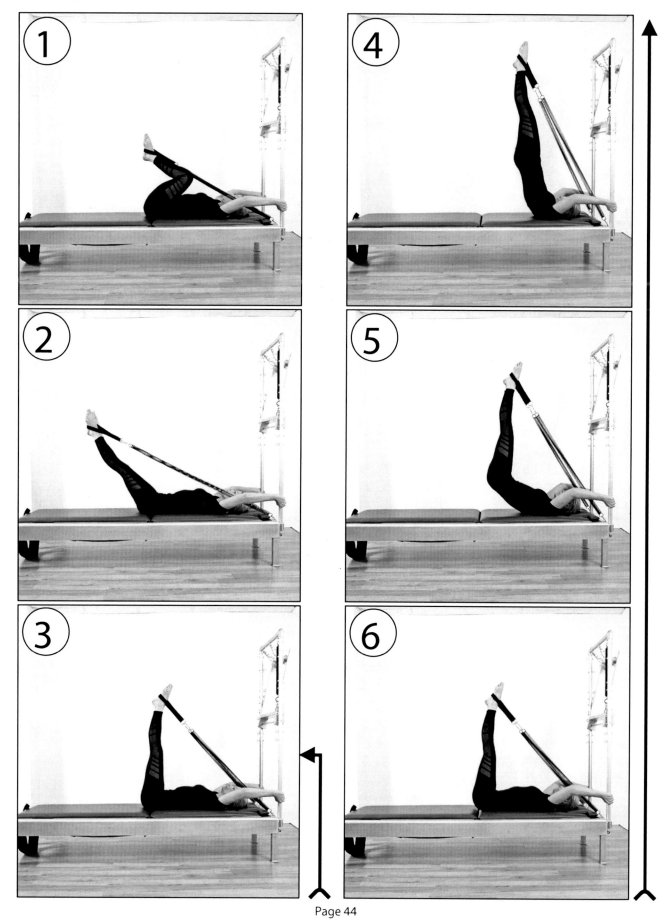

16. Reformer based Long Spine (M)
2/3

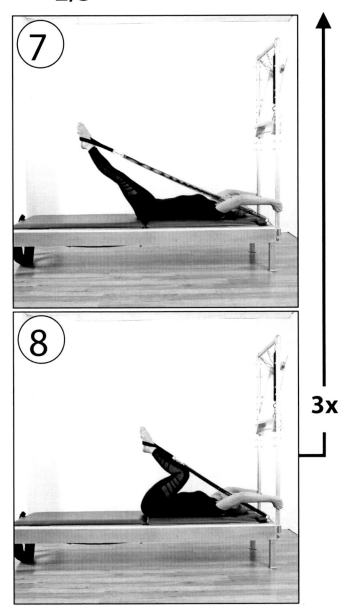

3x

16. Reformer based Long Spine (M)
3/3

Setup:
If possible, attach traditional leg springs at mat height. Supine position with the head pointing toward the spring attachments. The distance to the vertical bars of the Cadillac should be between half an arm-length and one arm-length. The hands hold the vertical bars slightly above the shoulders. Pelvis in a neutral position, spine in a natural position. Feet in the loops, the loops are in the arch of the foot, tendentially closer to the heels. When using double loops, pick up the larger loop to ease some of the pressure from the springs. The legs are parallel, feet stretched. Bend the legs with the knees as close to the body as comfortably possible. The feet are slightly above the knees.

Purpose of the Exercise:
Mobilization of the entire spine with the focus on the thoracic spine.

Execution: 3x - 5x
Image 2: Stretch the legs upward to approx. 45 degrees, the springs run just above the shoulders, not coming into contact with them. Initiate the stretch from the inner thighs. Shortly keep the legs stretched.
Image 3: Raise the legs to 90 degrees.
Image 4: Roll upward as far as possible while maintaining the vertical legs. Make sure to go only as far as possible without exerting any pressure on the cervical spine. Ideally, the head can be lifted just barely in this position.
Image 5-6: Roll down vertebra by vertebra, keeping the legs vertical.
Image 7: Bring the legs back to 45 degrees. Repeat 3x-5x.
Image 8: After the last repetition, bend the legs again.

Common Mistakes:
In images 2-5 the legs are transported backward too much by the springs. One is folded with the head flat on the knees. Instead take an active position, rounded with some space between the head and knees, like an inverted Teaser, so the lower back can extend. No stretch!
In images 6-7 the movement becomes imprecise and too fast due to the lack of spring support.
In images 4-6, too much pressure is exerted on the cervical spine.

Modifications or Variations:
The feet are in a small V, the legs slightly outward rotated.
Open the legs slightly in the vertical position (Image 4) and roll down with the legs still open. Bring the legs to 45 degrees and then close them again.

Contraindications/Risks:
The exercise causes an increased strain on the shoulder and should therefore only be performed by people with healthy shoulders.
In the overhead positions, make sure that the cervical spine is not overstrained.

17. X-Legs (M)

1/4 Alternative name: Lobster

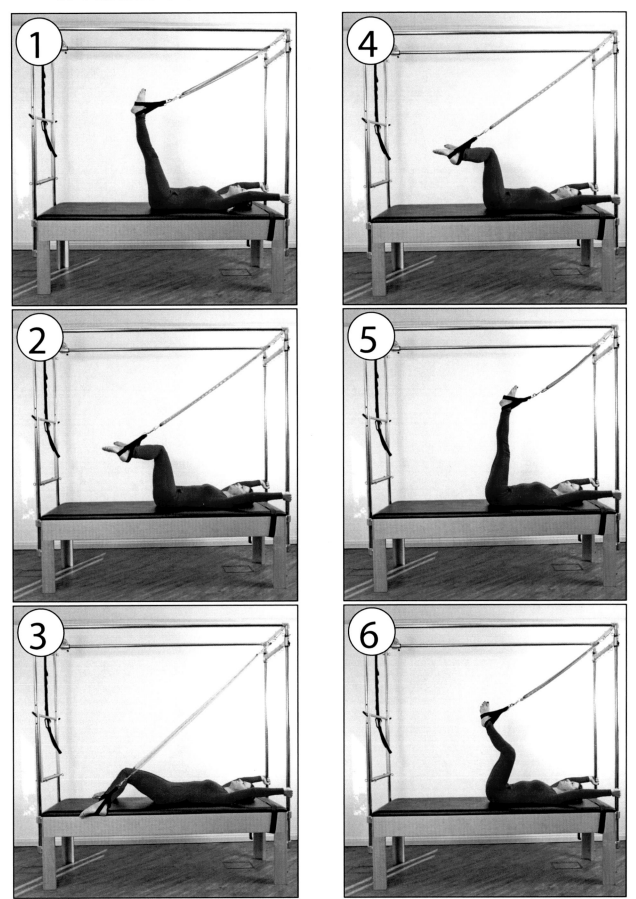

17. X-Legs (M)

2/4 Alternative name: Lobster

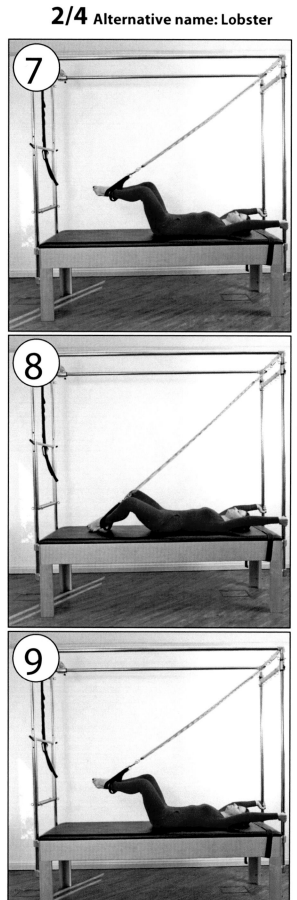

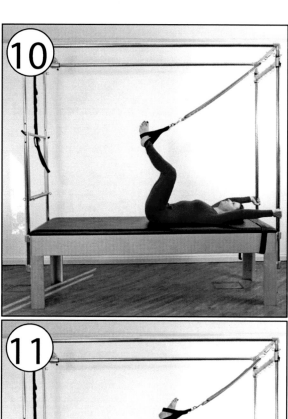

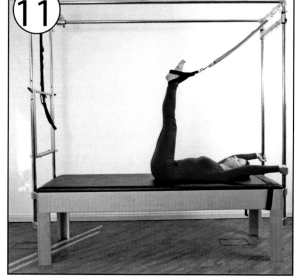

17. X-Legs (M)

3/4 Alternative name: Lobster

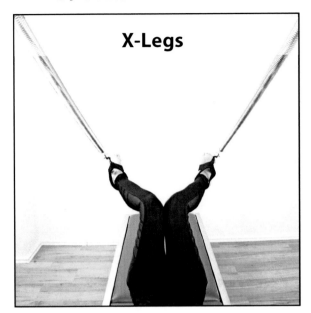

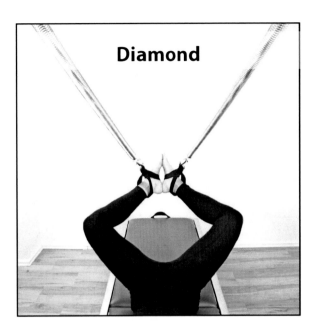

Setup:

Select the spring position so that the exercise can be performed completely and without any evasive movements. The height of the spring position also influences the effect of the exercise. Typically, the long, soft leg springs are attached at the highest possible point of the Cadillac. Ideally, use Y-loops or gyro-double-loops that run both along the arch and around the ankle of the foot.

Supine position with the head pointing toward the spring attachments. The distance to the vertical bars of the Cadillac should be between half an arm-length and one arm-length. The further away, the harder the exercise. The springs should not hang loosely when the legs are vertical. The hands hold the vertical bars slightly above the shoulders or lie alongside the body. Pelvis in a neutral position, spine in a natural position. The feet are in the loops. The legs are parallel, closed with inner tension and stretched out vertically. If the vertical position cannot be reached while maintaining a natural spinal position (danger of a posterior pelvic tilt and pressure on the lumbar spine), move the legs upward only as long as the hip remains stable. The feet are parallel and stretched.

Purpose of the Exercise:

Mobilization of the hip.
Strengthening of the internal and external leg rotators and feet muscles.
Moving the knees and feet at maximum internal and external rotation.
Decoupling the leg movement from the hip and torso.

17. X-Legs (M)

4/4 Alternative name: Lobster

Execution: 5x - 10x per side

Pull the abdomen inward and upward. Stabilize the entire trunk with the muscles.

Image 2:	Bend the knees and simultaneously rotate the legs inward. Slightly more than 90 degrees between the thighs and lower legs. X-leg position. The knees hold the forward tension. The big toes push outward. The thighs are vertical.
Image 3:	Maintain the angle of the thighs and lower the legs to the outer edge of the Cadillac or even outside the Cadillac. The tight knee position will automatically widen slightly.
Image 4:	Raise the legs back up as far as possible while maintaining the angle between thigh and lower leg. Hold the neutral pelvic position.
Image 5:	Then stretch the legs upward. The legs are parallel again. Now flex and point the feet (not shown in the images).
Image 6:	Fold the knees outward, bringing the legs into the diamond position. The soles of the feet lie on top of each other. The feet tilt away from the body (no leg movement yet), the toes do not point upwards but away from the body.
Image 7-8:	In the diamond position, lower the legs until the little toes touch - if possible - the Cadillac mat. Do not extend the legs.
Image 9-10:	Bring the legs back up into the diamond. The big toes still point as far away from the body as possible.
Image 11:	Stretch the legs upward. The legs are parallel. Now flex the feet (not shown in the images).

Common Mistakes:

The stability of the pelvis is neglected.
The feet sickle in the X-leg position (supination).
Instead of holding the forward tension in the X-leg position, the legs fall toward each other.
The movement in the diamond position is not led by the small toes.
The footwork is neglected in both positions.

Modifications or Variations:

From the deep X-leg position, do not raise the legs again but instead stretch them downward and rotate them outward. Come back up in a large circle. To change the direction, move the legs outward and downward. At the bottom, rotate the legs inward and bring the knees to the inside, back to the X-leg position. In this position, come back up and then stretch the legs upward.

Contraindications/Risks:

Danger of luxation in case of fresh hip endoprostheses.

18. Peter Pan (M)
1/2

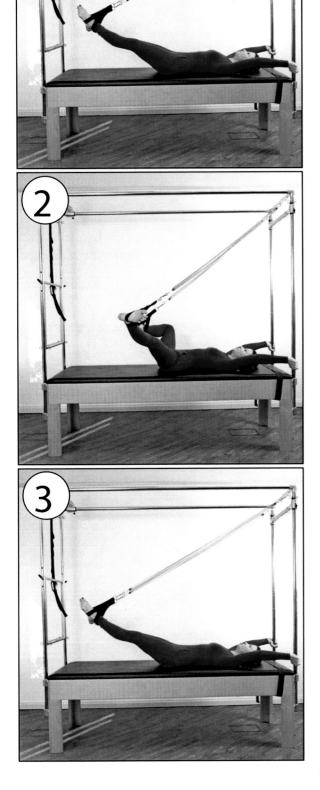

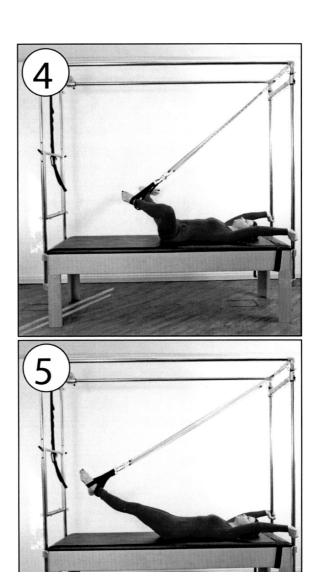

Alternative Perspective

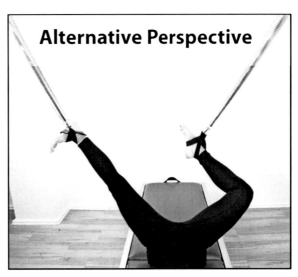

18. Peter Pan (M)
2/2

Setup:

Select the spring position so that the exercise can be performed completely and without any evasive movements. The height of the spring position also influences the effect of the exercise. Typically, the long, soft leg springs are attached at the highest possible point of the Cadillac. Ideally, use Y-loops or gyro-double-loops that run both along the arch and around the ankle of the foot.

Supine position with the head pointing toward the spring attachments. The distance to the vertical bars of the Cadillac should be between half an arm-length and one arm-length. The further away, the harder the exercise. The springs should not hang loosely when the legs are vertical. The hands hold the vertical bars slightly above the shoulders or lie alongside the body. Pelvis in a neutral position, spine in a natural position. The feet are in the loops. The legs are in a slight outward rotation, <u>feet in a small V</u> (heels together, toes apart) and stretched, closed with inner tension at 45 degrees or lower.

Purpose of the Exercise:

Mobilization of the hip.
Stretch of the inner thighs.
Decoupling the leg movement from the hip and torso.

Execution: 5x - 7x per side

Pull the abdomen inward and upward. Stabilize the entire trunk with the muscles.
The right leg is bent and the knee pulls the thigh to the right. The right foot is stretched on the way to the end position and points to the left. At the same time, the left leg is stretched and moved outward. During the movement, the left foot is flexed.
Both feet are at the same height. Open until a slight stretch is reached across both inner thighs.
Bring both legs back together, into the starting position.
Now the left leg is bent and the knee pulls the thigh to the left. The left foot is stretched on the way to the end position and points to the right. At the same time, the right leg is stretched and moved outward. During the movement, the right foot is flexed.
Both feet are at the same height. Open until a slight stretch is reached across both inner thighs.
Bring both legs back together, into the starting position.

Common Mistakes:

The pelvis swings along toward the side of the stretched leg.
The bent knee does not pull to the side but is kept in the center.
The feet move at different heights.
The bent leg is too passive.
One forgets to move the legs back to the center half-way through the movement.
The foot positions are not fully assumed.
The foot that is stretched sickles (supination). The foot that is flexed is not sufficiently pulled toward the knee with the edge of the small toe.

Modifications or Variations:

The pelvis swings along toward the side of the stretched leg. The hips remain lowered.

Contraindications/Risks:

Danger of luxation in case of fresh hip endoprostheses through the outward rotation in combination with abduction.

19. Windmill (M)
1/4

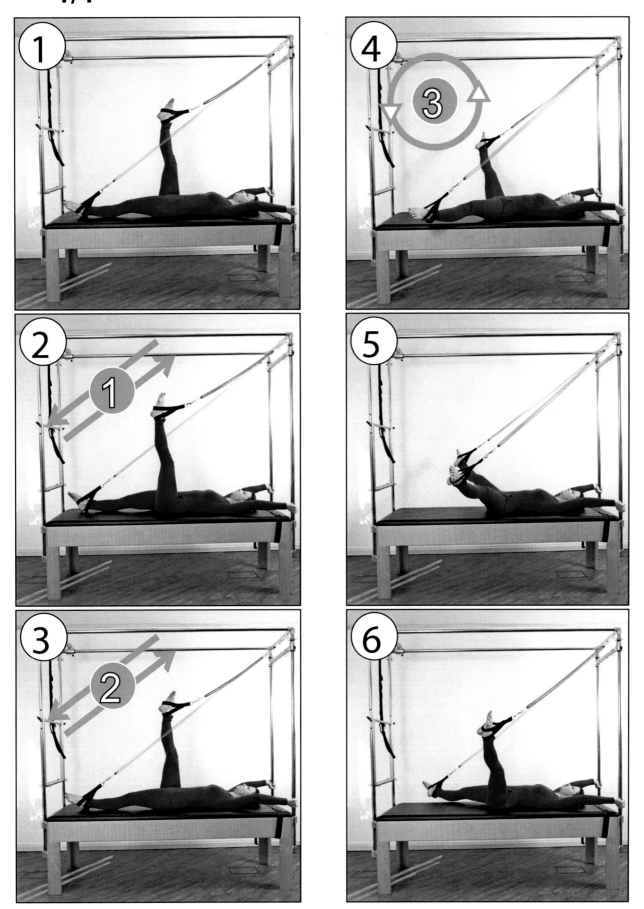

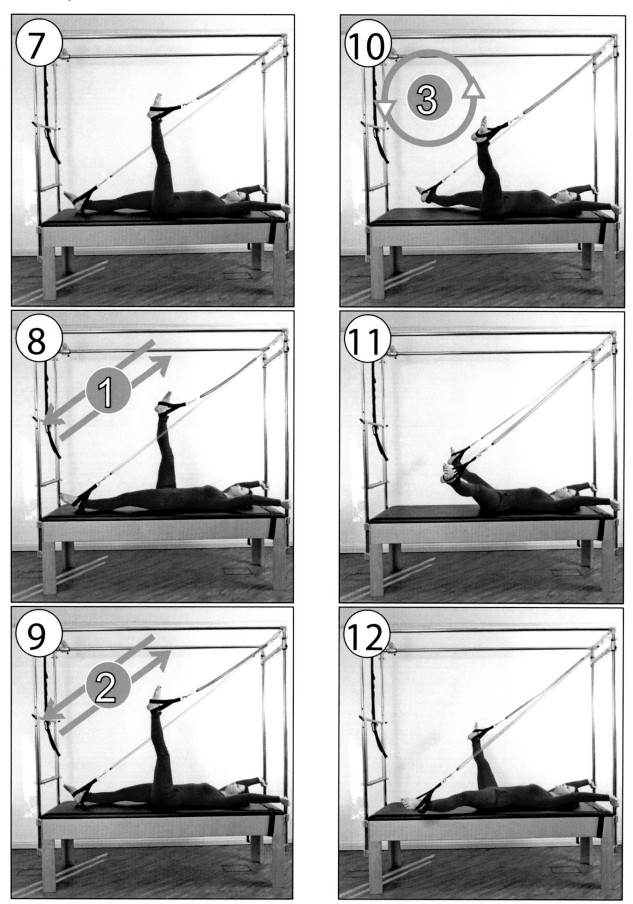

19. Windmill (M)
3/4

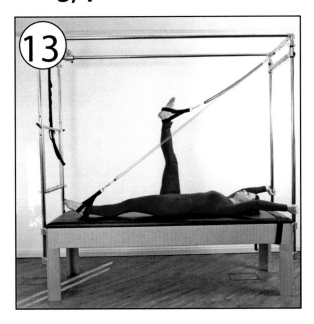

Setup:

Select the spring position so that the exercise can be performed completely and without any evasive movements. The height of the spring position also influences the effect of the exercise. Typically, the long, soft leg springs are attached at the highest possible point of the Cadillac. Ideally, use Y-loops or gyro-double-loops that run both along the arch and around the ankle of the foot.

Supine position with the head pointing toward the spring attachments. The distance to the vertical bars of the Cadillac should be between half an arm-length and one arm-length. The further away, the harder the exercise. The springs should not hang loosely when the legs are vertical. The hands hold the vertical bars slightly above the shoulders or lie alongside the body. Pelvis in a neutral position, spine in a natural position. The feet are in the loops. The legs are parallel, closed with inner tension and stretched out vertically. If the vertical position cannot be reached while maintaining a natural spinal position (danger of a posterior pelvic tilt and pressure on the lumbar spine), move the legs upward only as long as the hip remains stable. The feet are parallel and stretched.

Purpose of the Exercise:

Mobilization of the hip.
Strengthening of the hip and knee extensors.
Decoupling the leg movement from the hip and torso.
Stretch of the leg backsides and inner thighs.
Improvement of the coordinative abilities.

19. Windmill (M)
4/4

Execution: 6x - 10x

Pull the abdomen inward and upward. Stabilize the entire trunk with the muscles.

Image 1:   With the foot stretched, lower the left leg toward the Cadillac mat, without otherwise changing the body position. Viewed from the side, the end position looks like a capital "L" with one leg stretched upward and one laid down. This is the starting position.

Image 2:   1. Switch
Bring the upward-stretched right leg downward. Simultaneously, raise the left leg into the "L".

Image 3:   2. Switch
Now lower the left leg and raise the right one.

Image 4-7:   3. Windmill
Move the right leg further to the right side and lower it in a half-circle until it is completely laid down. Simultaneously, bring the left leg further to the left and raise it in a half-circle until it is stretched up.

Image 8:   1. Switch
Bring the upward-stretched left leg downward. Simultaneously, raise the right leg into the "L".

Image 8:   2. Switch
Now lower the right leg and raise the left one.

Image 10-13:   3. Windmill
Move the left leg further to the left side and lower it in a half-circle until it is completely laid down. Simultaneously, bring the right leg further to the right and raise it in a half-circle until it is stretched up.

Common Mistakes:

The stability of the pelvis is neglected.
The feet sickle (supination) in the extension and the flexion.
The windmill-movement is performed imprecisely or even incorrectly.

Modifications or Variations:

If the coordination of the windmill movement is overwhelming, do not move your legs at the same time but one by one. For example, first move the upper leg down in a semicircle and then the lower leg up in a semicircle.

To make the exercise more demanding in terms of coordination, alternately flex and stretch the feet during the "scissor movements". For example, come up in a flex and down in a point. The windmill movement is then also performed completely with both feet flexed.

Execution with a "Helicopter", i.e. turning 5x into one direction and then 5x into the other direction.

Contraindications/Risks:

Danger of luxation in case of fresh hip endoprostheses through the outward rotation of the legs.

20. One Leg Cross Spring Series (T)
1/6

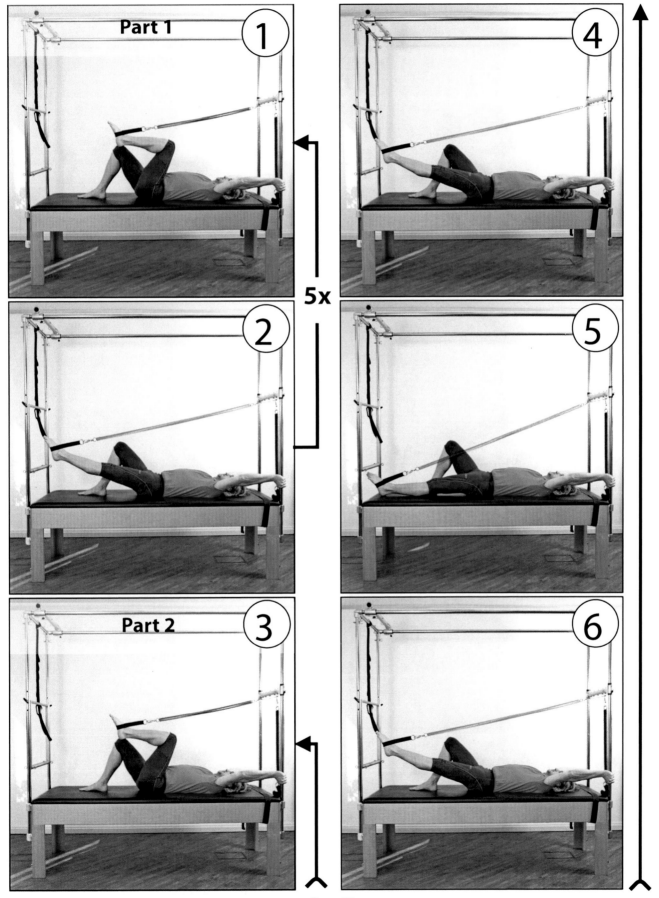

20. One Leg Cross Spring Series (T)
2/6

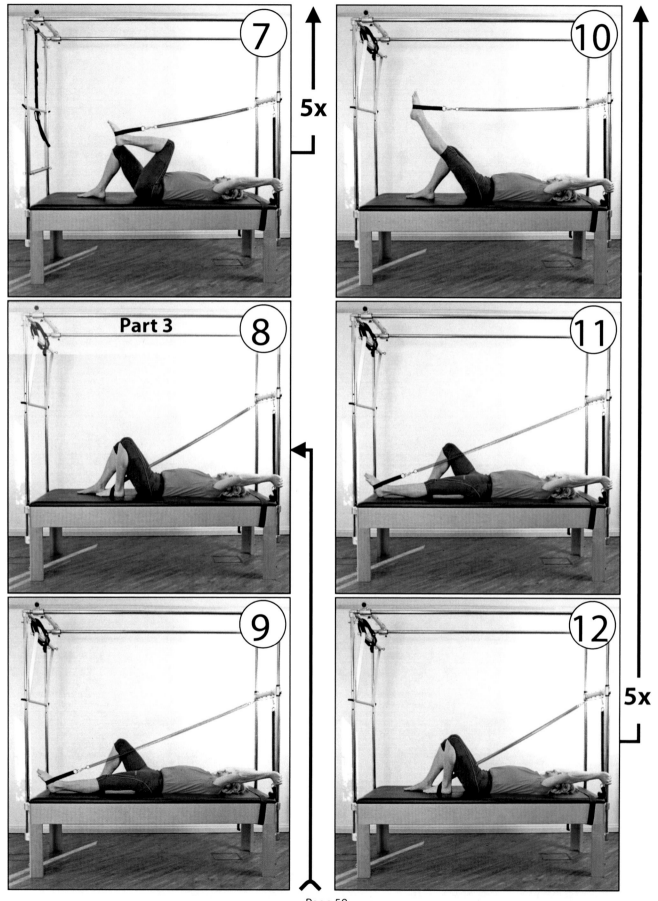

Part 3

20. One Leg Cross Spring Series (T)
3/6

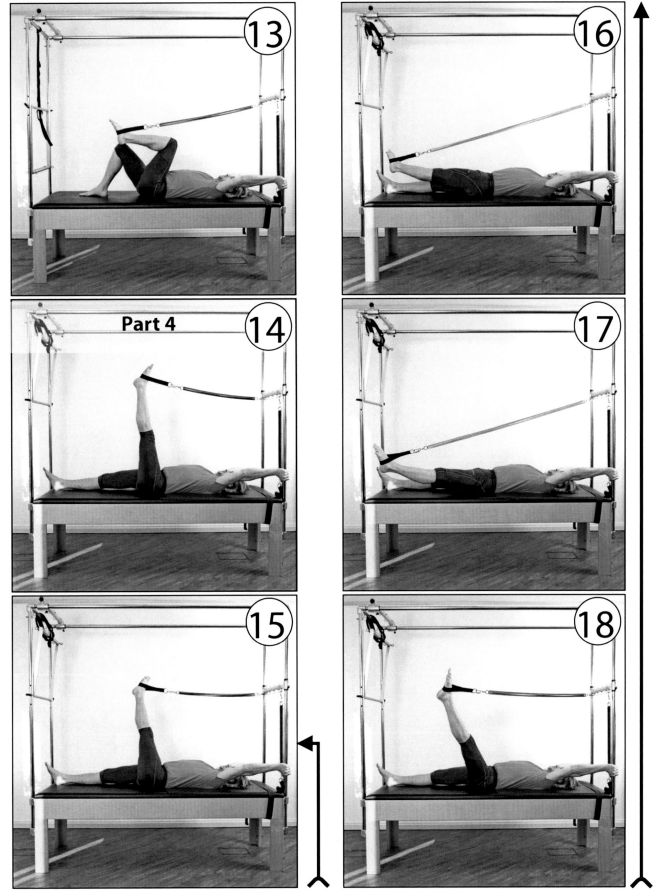

20. One Leg Cross Spring Series (T)
4/6

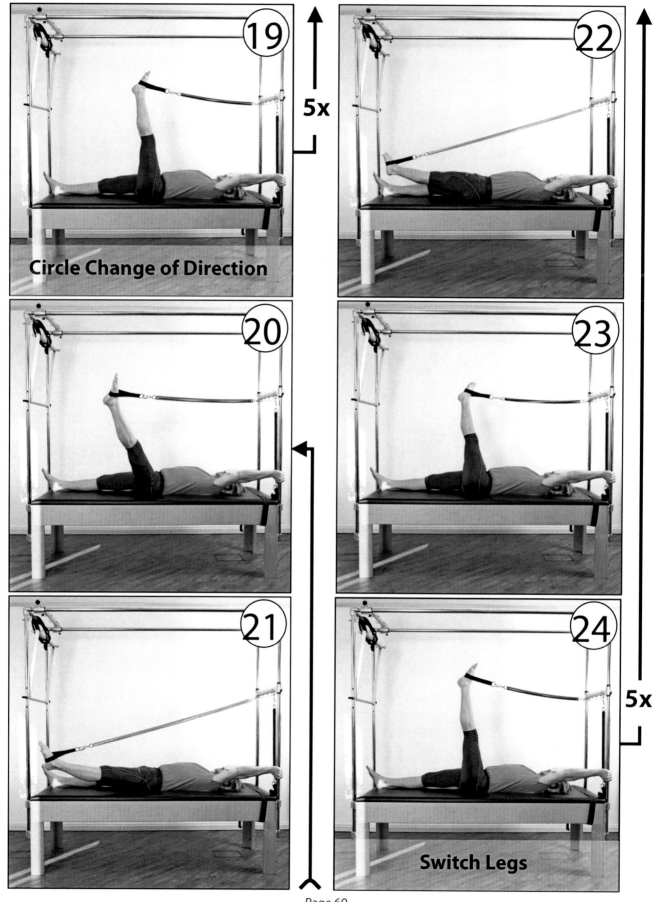

Circle Change of Direction

5x

Switch Legs

5x

20. One Leg Cross Spring Series (T)
5/6

Setup:

Attach traditional leg springs at a height of 80 - 85 cm / 31.5 - 33.5 inches. The higher the spring attachment, the more the leg backsides have to work.

Supine position with the head pointing toward the spring attachments. The distance to the vertical bars of the Cadillac should be between half an arm-length and one arm-length. The further away, the harder the exercise. The hands hold the vertical bars slightly above the shoulders. Pelvis in a neutral position, spine in a natural position. <u>Left foot in the loop of the right spring.</u> The loops are in the arch of the foot with a tendency toward the heel. The right leg is bent, the feet stands on the Cadillac mat. The left foot is on the same height as the right knee.

Purpose of the Exercise:

Strengthening of the leg and knee stabilizers with the focus on the outer leg side.

Execution: repetitions as described below

Pull the abdomen inward and upward. Stabilize the entire trunk with the muscles.

Part 1 - Image 1-2:
Stretch the left leg so that the left foot is brought forward, remaining at the same height. Bend the left leg until the left foot is parallel to the right knee again. When stretching forward and bending backward, the foot, shin and knee always move on a line that is parallel to the outer edge of the Cadillac.
Repeat 5x.

Part 2 - Image 3-7:
Stretch the left leg so that the left foot is brought forward, remaining at the same height. Lay the left leg down on the mat, still stretched, and raise it again until the left foot is at the same height as the right knee. Bend the left leg until the left foot is parallel to the right knee again. When stretching forward and bending backward, the foot, shin and knee always move on a line that is parallel to the outer edge of the Cadillac.
Repeat 5x.

Part 3 - Image 8-12:
Bend the left leg and place the left foot on the mat. The spring runs between the legs. Stretch the left leg out on the mat. Raise the left leg until the left knee is on the height of the right knee. Stretch the leg out on the mat again. Bend the left leg again, pulling the foot toward the buttocks. The spring runs between the legs.
Repeat 5x.

Part 4 - Image 13-14:
Raise the left leg and stretch it upward vertically. Simultaneously, stretch the right leg out on the mat.

Image 15-19:
Via the center of the body, move the left leg to the right. Throughout the movement, the pelvis remains stable. In a circle, bring the leg to the right foot and further to the left outer edge. Then bring it back to the vertical pole.
Repeat 5x.

Image 20-24: Bring the left leg to the left as long as the pelvis still lies completely stable. Then lower the leg toward the right foot in a circle. Finally, bring it to the right pole via the center of the body.
Repeat 5x.

Switch legs.

20. One Leg Cross Spring Series (T)
6/6

Common Mistakes:

The knee is unstable and swings around while moving.
The foot is not kept at knee height during Part 1 and 2.
The leg is moved upward without stopping instead of moving just up to knee height.
The pelvis is rotated or pulled upward on one side.

Modifications or Variations:

For very tall people, the use of an additional carabiner can lengthen the leg springs so that the force at the end of the movement is not too great.
The hands lie down at the sides of the body.

Contraindications/Risks:

Danger of luxation in case of fresh hip endoprostheses through the outward rotation of the legs. Hence, omit the last part of the exercise.

21. One Leg Diagonal Bicylce (M)
   1/4

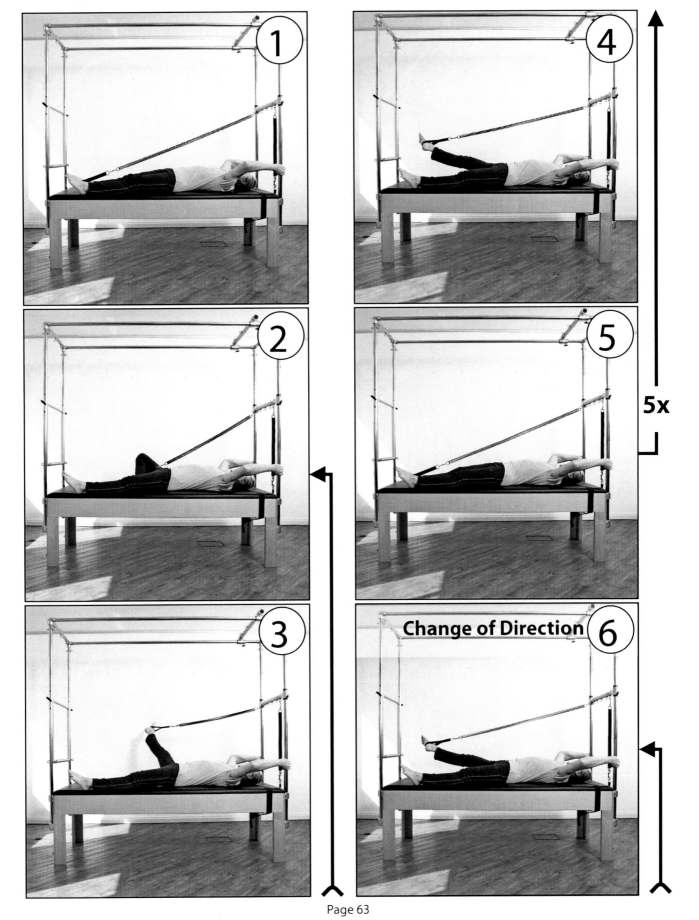

21. One Leg Diagonal Bicycle (M)
   2/4

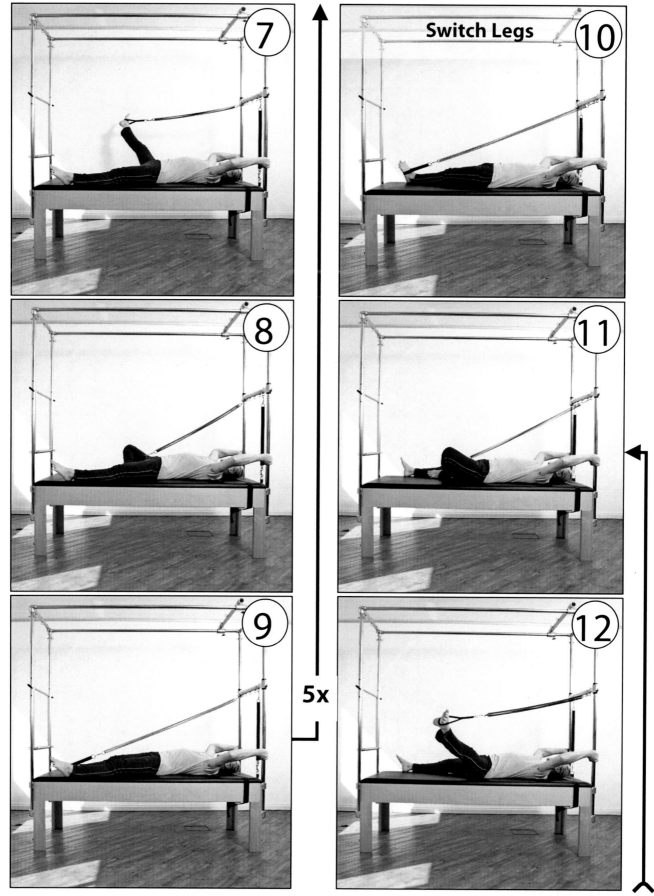

21. One Leg Diagonal Bicycle (M)
3/4

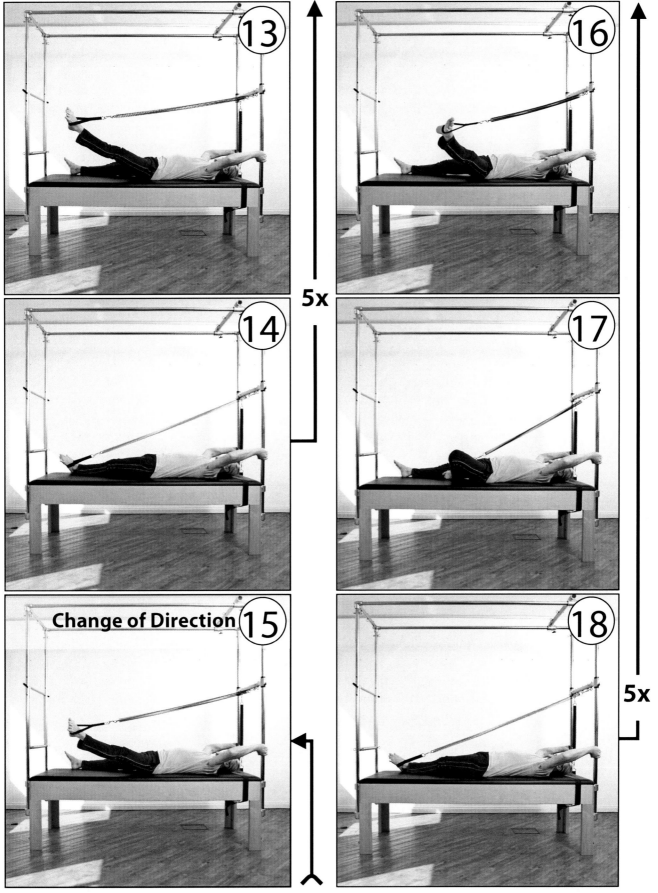

13

14

Change of Direction 15

5x

16

17

18

5x

21. One Leg Diagonal Bicycle (M)
4/4

Setup:

Attach traditional leg springs at a height of 80 - 85 cm / 31.5 - 33.5 inches. The higher the spring attachment, the more the leg backsides have to work.

Supine position with the head pointing toward the spring attachments. The distance to the vertical bars of the Cadillac should be between half an arm-length and one arm-length. The further away, the harder the exercise. The hands hold the vertical bars slightly above the shoulders. Pelvis in a neutral position, spine in a natural position.

<u>Right foot</u> in the loop of <u>the right spring</u>. The loops are in the arch of the foot with a tendency toward the heel. Stretch the left leg and bring it to the left side until the heel touches the left edge of the mat. The right leg lies next to the left one. Both feet are stretched in a small V.

Purpose of the Exercise:

Strengthening of the leg and knee stabilizers with the focus on the inner thighs.

Stabilization of the multifidus, transversus abdominis, pelvic floor musculature, internal and external oblique and the rectus abdomis.

Execution:

Pull the abdomen inward and upward. Stabilize the entire trunk with the muscles.

Image 2:   Bend the right leg and bring the right foot to the inner side of the left foot ankle. Meanwhile, move the right knee outward. The right foot slightly strokes the inner side of the left lower and upper leg.

Image 3:   When the foot cannot be pulled any further, stretch the right leg outward diagonally. Only move the right leg outward as far as the pelvis can still lie down without moving.

Image 4-5:   Stretch the right leg while lowering it in a straight line toward the left leg. The legs now lie next to each other.

Repeat 5x, then change the direction.

Image 6-7:   Move the stretched right leg to the right side in a straight, diagonal line. Only move the right leg outward so far as the pelvis can still lie on the mat without moving.

Image 8-9:   Bend the right leg with the knee pointing out to the side. Starting from above, move the right foot along the inside of the left upper and then lower thigh to the foot ankle and finally lay it down until it lies next to the left leg, stretched out.

Repeat 5x, then switch legs.

Common Mistakes:

The leg is moved too far to the side, causing the pelvis to rotate and be pulled upward on one side.
The moving leg is not lied down next to the other completely at the beginning and end of every movement.
Lack of an outward rotation in both legs.

Modifications or Variations:

For very tall people, the use of an additional carabiner can lengthen the leg springs so that the force at the end of the movement is not too great.
The hands are laid down down sideways next to the body.

Contraindications/Risks:

Danger of luxation in case of fresh hip endoprostheses through the outward rotation of the legs. Hence, omit the last part of the exercise.

22. Pull Down Side Lying (T)
1/2

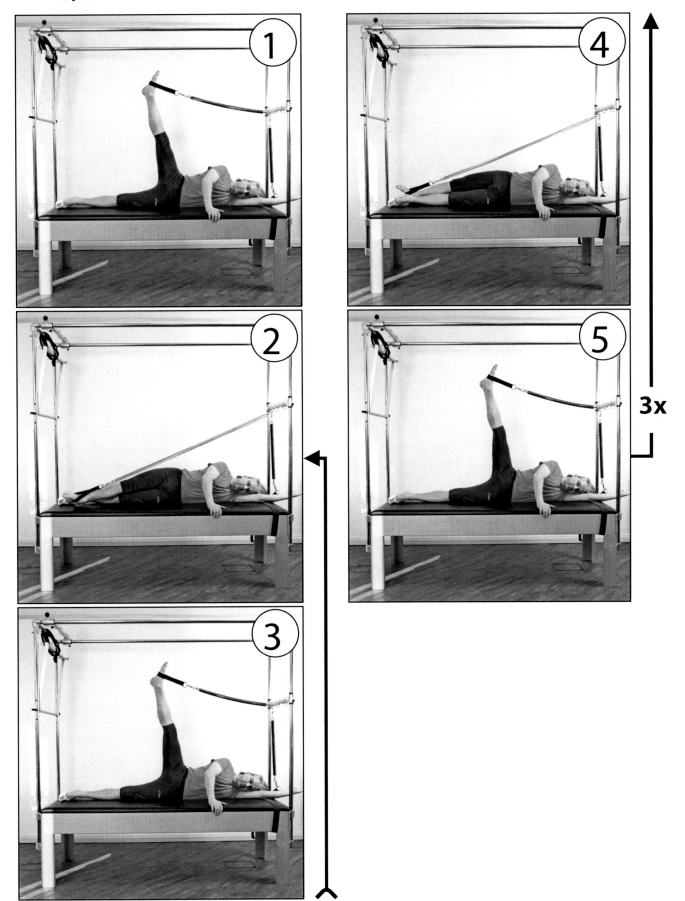

1

4

2

3

5

3x

22. **Pull Down Side Lying (T)**
2/2

Setup:

Attach traditional leg springs at a height of 80 - 85 cm / 31.5 - 33.5 inches. The higher the spring attachment, the more the leg backsides and inner thighs have to work.

If possible, attach the spring centrally. In case a central attachment of the leg spring is used, lie in a lateral position in the center of the mat with the head pointing toward the spring attachments. If the central attachment is not possible, lie on the back edge of the Cadillac with the leg backsides, buttocks, back and head (Caution! Risk of falling) and use the spring on this side. In both cases, the body forms a straight line when viewed from above. Pelvis in a neutral position, spine in a natural position. The distance to the vertical bars of the Cadillac should be between half an arm-length and one arm-length. The further away, the harder the exercise.

When lying at the edge at half an arm-length distance, bring the elbow and forearm toward the vertical bar of the Cadillac. For a full arm-length, bring the hand of the lower arm toward the vertical bar of the Cadillac and push away from it. In both cases, bring the upper arm forward and place it on the mat in front of the chest for support. The foot of the upper leg is in the loop. The loop is in the arch of the foot with a tendency toward the heel. The upper leg is stretched upward in an outward rotation. <u>The foot is stretched.</u>

Purpose of the Exercise:

Strengthening of the leg backsides and inner thighs, as well as the external leg rotators.
Mobilization of the hip joint.

Execution: 5x - 10x per side

Pull the abdomen inward and upward. Stabilize the entire trunk with the muscles.

Image 2:   In the outward rotation, lower the upper, stretched leg.
                 The upper foot touches the Cadillac mat directly in front of the lower foot with its heel.
Image 3:   Bring the leg back into the starting position.
Image 4:   In the outward rotation, lower the upper, stretched leg. The upper foot touches the Cadillac mat directly behind the lower foot with its heel (or, if lying at the outer edge of the Cadillac, stop the downward movement in the air, right behind the lower foot).
Image 5:   Bring the leg back into the starting position.

Repeat 5x - 10x, then switch sides.

Common Mistakes:

Viewed from above, there is no straight line. Usually, the torso and now sunk-in head are slightly tilted forward instead of remaining in one line with the leg on the mat.
The outward rotation of the leg is not held and the foot, therefore, does not point upward.

Modifications or Variations:

Instead of coming down in front of and behind the lower foot with the upper one, stretch the upper leg along the lower one. Extension.
For very tall people, the use of an additional carabiner can lengthen the leg springs so that the force at the end of the movement is not too great.
Instead of switching sides, immediately continue with the "Side Kick" and/or other exercises.
Attach long, soft leg springs at a higher point on the Cadillac, if possible with Y-loops or gyro-double-loops that run both along the arch and around the ankle of the foot.
Move the lower leg forward for more stability.

Contraindications/Risks:

Danger of luxation in case of fresh hip endoprostheses.

23. Side Kick (T)
1/3

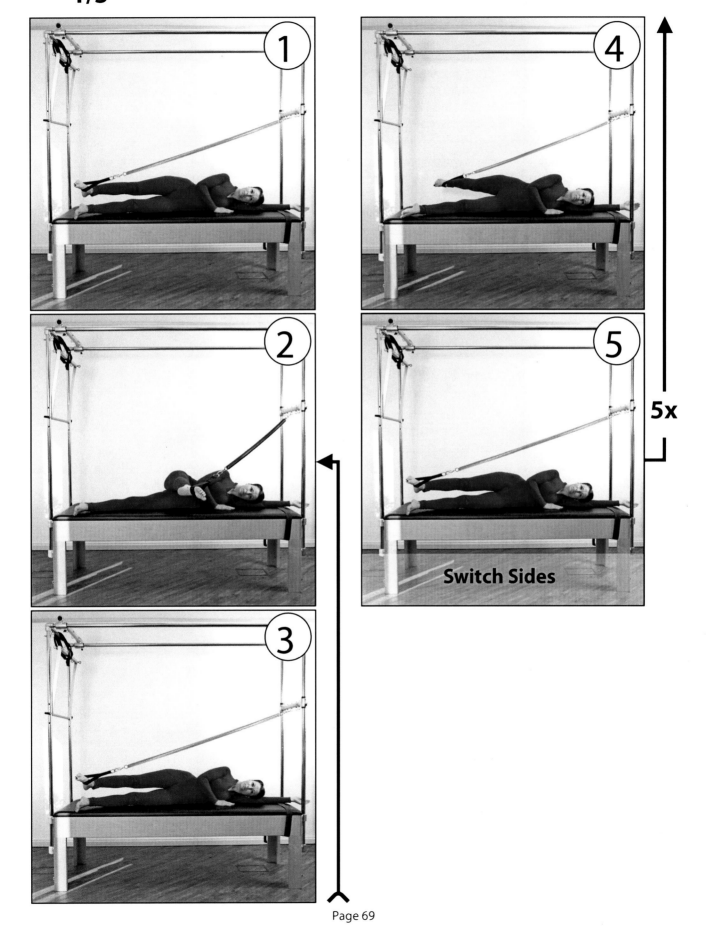

Switch Sides

5x

23. Side Kick (T)
2/3

Setup:

Attach traditional leg springs at a height of 80 - 85 cm / 31.5 - 33.5 inches. The higher the spring attachment, the more the leg backsides and inner thighs have to work.

If possible, attach the spring centrally. In case a central attachment of the leg spring is used, lie in a lateral position in the center of the mat with the head pointing toward the spring attachments. If the central attachment is not possible, lie on the back edge of the Cadillac with the leg backsides, buttocks, back and head (Caution! risk of falling) and use the spring on this side.

In both cases bring the lower leg forward as far as possible with the lower foot still lying on the Cadillac mat. The rest of the body forms a straight line when viewed from above. Pelvis in a neutral position, spine in a natural position. The distance to the vertical bars of the Cadillac should be between half an arm-length and one arm-length. The further away, the harder the exercise.

When lying at the edge at half an arm-length distance, bring the elbow and forearm toward the vertical bar of the Cadillac. For a full arm-length, bring the hand of the lower arm toward the vertical bar of the Cadillac and push away from it.

In both cases, bring the upper arm forward and place it on the mat in front of the chest for support.

The foot of the upper leg is in the loop. The loop is in the arch of the foot with a tendency toward the heel. The upper leg is stretched upward in a slight outward rotation. <u>The foot is stretched.</u>

Purpose of the Exercise:

Decoupling the leg movement from the hip and torso.
Stretch of the deep hip flexors and slight stretch of the leg backsides.
Mobilization of the hip joint.
Strengthening of the gluteal musculature through the outward rotation.
Slight strengthening of the inner thighs.

Execution: 5x - 10x per side

Pull the abdomen inward and upward. Stabilize the entire trunk with the muscles.

Image 2: With the leg and foot in a slight outward rotation, stretch the foot forward as far as possible without changing the body position.

Image 3: Bring the leg back into the starting position.

Image 4: Pull the abdomen inward and upward. Without pausing, move the upper, stretched leg backward as far as possible without otherwise changing the body position. The leg and foot are parallel.

Image 5: Bring the leg back into the starting position.

Repeat 5x - 10x, then change the direction.

Keep the pelvis as stable as possible, while, nonetheless, letting it react and move naturally into both directions. However, let neither the pelvis, nor the torso rotate forward or backward. Furthermore, there is no compression of the lumbar spine in the extension. Therefore, particularly make sure to pull the abdominal muscles inward to protect the lower back.

23. Side Kick (T)
3/3

Common Mistakes:

Viewed from above, there is no straight line. Usually, the torso and now sunk-in head are slightly tilted forward instead of remaining in one line with the leg on the mat.

The leg alternates in height on the way forward and backward.

The torso swings forward during the leg's backward movement to compensate for the movement.

The back is rounded during the forward leg movement. The leg is moved too far back during the backward movement, which causes a hollow back.

The iliac spines (spina iliaca anterior superior) do not lie on top of each other, instead the upper edge of the pelvis is closer to the lowest rib.

The foot of the upper leg sickles (supination).

Modifications or Variations:

For very tall people, the use of an additional carabiner can lengthen the leg springs so that the force at the end of the movement is not too great.

Rotate the upper leg outward instead of keeping it in a parallel position. Typically, this reduces the backward movement.

When kicking forward, flex the foot and remain in the end position for a second, then kick again and move the leg slightly further. On the way back, stretch the foot. Do not repeat this a second time. Inner voice forward: kick, kick. Backward: Stretch.

Keep the pelvis completely stable. This will reduce the radius of motion.

Instead of switching sides, continue with the "Side Bicycle" and/or other exercises.

Attach long, soft leg springs at a higher point on the Cadillac, if possible with Y-loops or gyro-double-loops that run both along the arch and around the ankle of the foot.

To make the exercise more difficult, bring the lower leg into one straight line with the rest of the body.

Contraindications/Risks:

Danger of luxation in case of fresh hip endoprostheses.

24. Side Bicycle (T)
1/4

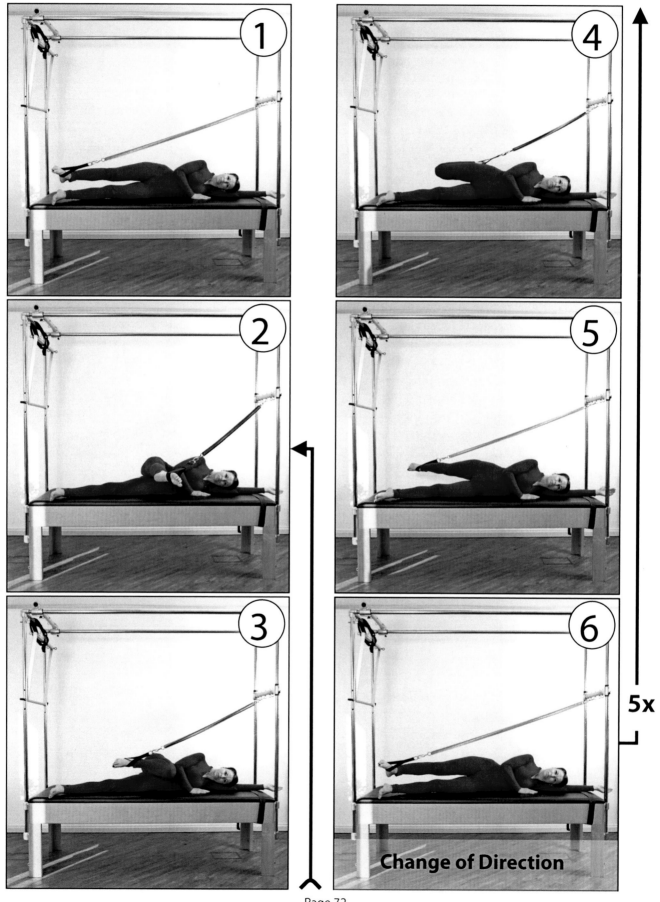

1

2

3

4

5

6

5x

Change of Direction

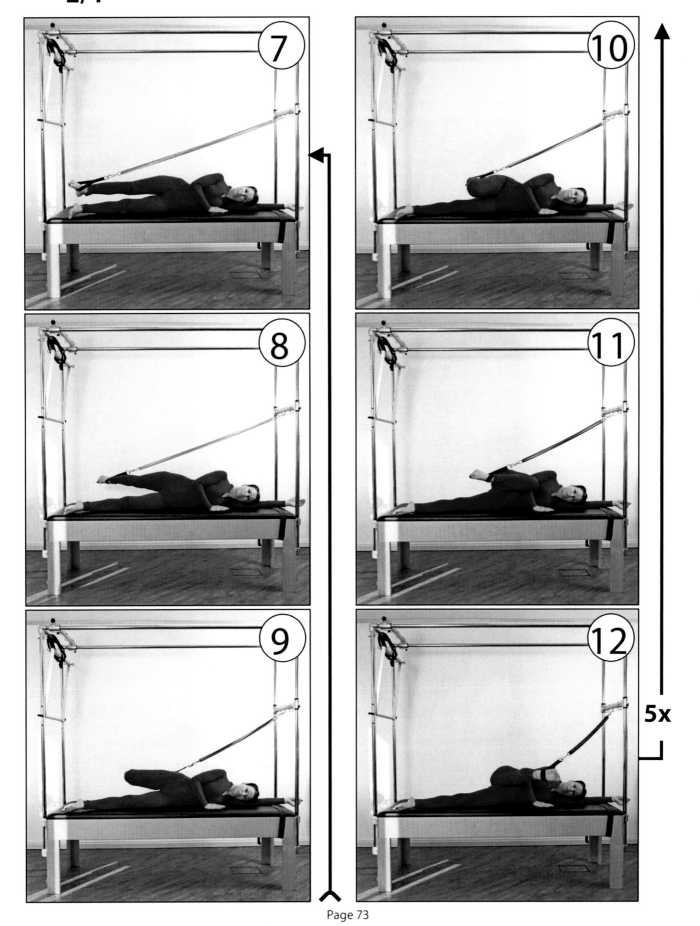

24. Side Bicycle (T)
3/4

Setup:

Attach traditional leg springs at a height of 80 - 85 cm / 31.5 - 33.5 inches. The higher the spring attachment, the more the leg backsides and inner thighs have to work.

If possible, attach the spring centrally. In case a central attachment of the leg spring is used, lie in a lateral position in the center of the mat with the head pointing toward the spring attachments. If the central attachment is not possible, lie on the back edge of the Cadillac with the leg backsides, buttocks, back and head (Caution! Risk of falling) and use the spring on this side.

In both cases bring the lower leg forward as far as possible with the lower foot still lying on the Cadillac mat. The rest of the body forms a straight line when viewed from above. Pelvis in a neutral position, spine in a natural position. The distance to the vertical bars of the Cadillac should be between half an arm-length and one arm-length. The further away, the harder the exercise.

When lying at the edge at half an arm-length distance, bring the elbow and forearm toward the vertical bar of the Cadillac. For a full arm-length, bring the hand of the lower arm toward the vertical bar of the Cadillac and push away from it. In both cases, bring the upper arm forward and place it on the mat in front of the chest for support. The foot of the upper leg is in the loop. The loop is in the arch of the foot with a tendency toward the heel. The upper leg is stretched upward in a slight outward rotation. <u>The foot is stretched.</u>

Purpose of the Exercise:

Stretch of the deep hip flexors and slight stretch of the leg backsides.
Mobilization of the hip joint.
Strengthening of the gluteal musculature through the outward rotation.
Slight strengthening of the inner thighs.

Execution: 5x - 10x per side

Pull the abdomen inward and upward. Stabilize the entire trunk with the muscles.

Image 2: Stretch the upper leg forward as far as possible without otherwise changing the body position. Ideally, maintain the slight outward rotation.

Image 3: Bend the knee and bring it as close to the chest as possible. Bring the foot to the buttocks while keeping the knee in the same place. Do not yet move it further backward.

Image 4: Only now, move the knee as far back as possible without otherwise moving the body.

Image 5: Pull the abdomen inward and upward. Without pausing, stretch the upper leg backward vertically. If possible, move the leg backward even further than the initial knee position. The leg and foot position is parallel.

Image 6: Bring the leg back into the starting position. Then bring the leg and foot into a slight external rotation.

Repeat 5x - 10x, then change the direction.

Image 7-8: Pull the abdomen in and upward, stretch the upper leg backward as far as possible without otherwise changing the body position and thereby falling into a hollow back. Foot is parallel.

Image 9: Bend the knee and bring the foot the foot to the buttocks, keeping the knee in the same place. Do not yet move it further backward.

Image 10-11: Staying as close as possible to the buttocks, bring the bent knee and foot forward and pull them as close as possible to the upper body. Do not round the back.

Image 12: Bring the leg as close as possible toward the head without otherwise changing the body position. Leg and foot are in a slight outward rotation.

Image 7: Bring the leg back into the starting position.

24. Side Bicycle (T)
4/4

Keep the pelvis as stable as possible, while, nonetheless, letting it react and move naturally into both directions. However, let neither the pelvis, nor the torso rotate forward or backward. Furthermore, there is no compression of the lumbar spine in the extension of the leg toward the hip or in the rounding with the leg flexed toward the hip. Therefore, particularly make sure to pull the abdominal muscles inward to protect the lower back.

Common Mistakes:

Viewed from above, there is no straight line. Usually, the torso and now sunk-in head are slightly tilted forward instead of remaining in one line with the leg on the mat.
The leg alternates in height on the way forward and backward.
The torso swings forward during the leg's backward movement to compensate for the movement. The back is rounded during the leg's forward movement.
The leg is moved too far back during the backward movement, which causes a hollow back.
The iliac spines (spina iliaca anterior superior) do not lie on top of each other, instead the upper edge of the pelvis is closer to the lowest rib.
The foot of the upper leg sickles (supination).

Modifications or Variations:

For very tall people, the use of an additional carabiner can lengthen the leg springs so that the force at the end of the movement is not too great.
Keep the pelvis completely stable. This will reduce the radius of motion.
Instead of switching sides, continue with the "Ronde de Jambe" and/or other exercises.
Attach long, soft leg springs at a higher point on the Cadillac, if possible with Y-loops or gyro-double-loops that run both along the arch and around the ankle of the foot.
To make the exercise more difficult, bring the lower leg into one straight line with the rest of the body.

Contraindications/Risks:

Danger of luxation in case of fresh hip endoprostheses.

25. Ronde de Jambe (T)

1/4 Alternative name: Side Lying Big Leg Circles

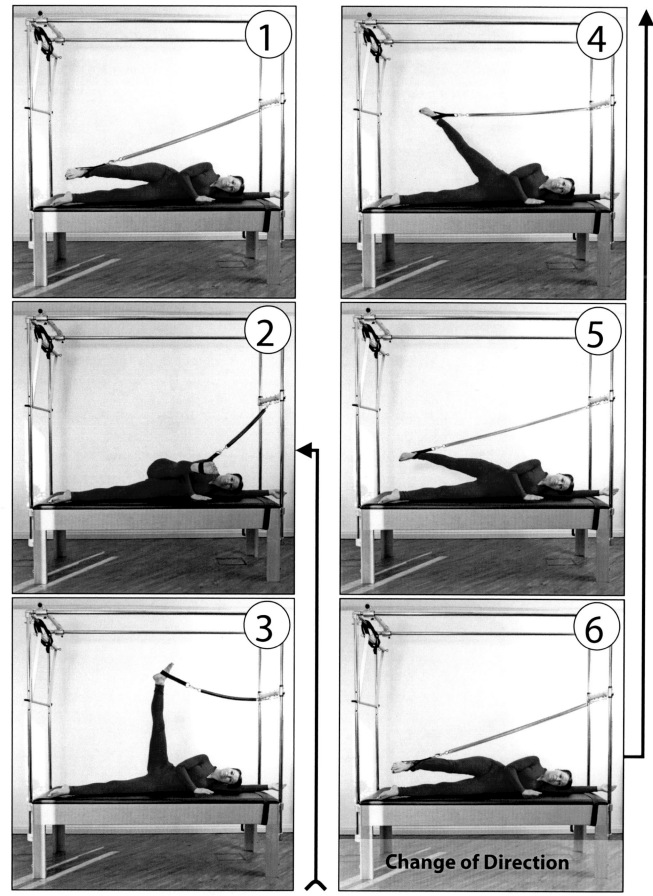

Change of Direction

25. Ronde de Jambe (T)

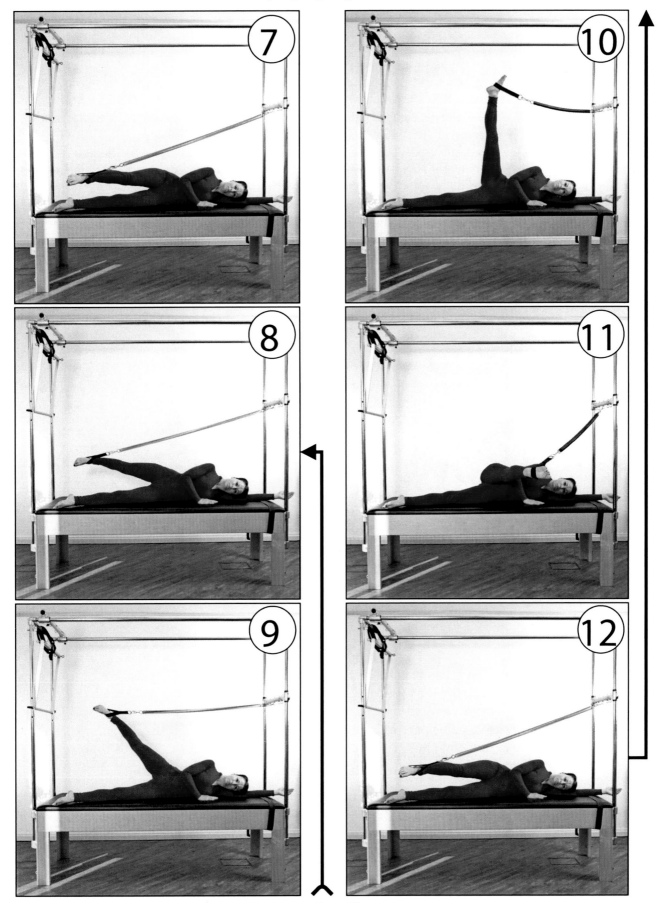

25. Ronde de Jambe (T)

3/4 Alternative name: Side Lying Big Leg Circles

Setup:

Attach traditional leg springs at a height of 80 - 85 cm / 31.5 - 33.5 inches. The higher the spring attachment, the more the leg backsides and inner thighs have to work.

If possible, attach the spring centrally. In case a central attachment of the leg spring is used, lie in a lateral position in the center of the mat with the head pointing toward the spring attachments. If the central attachment is not possible, lie on the back edge of the Cadillac with the leg backsides, buttocks, back and head (Caution! Risk of falling) and use the spring on this side.

In both cases bring the lower leg forward as far as possible with the lower foot still lying on the Cadillac mat. The rest of the body forms a straight line when viewed from above. Pelvis in a neutral position, spine in a natural position. The distance to the vertical bars of the Cadillac should be between half an arm-length and one arm-length. The further away, the harder the exercise.

When lying at the edge at half an arm-length distance, bring the elbow and forearm toward the vertical bar of the Cadillac. For a full arm-length, bring the hand of the lower arm toward the vertical bar of the Cadillac and push away from it.

In both cases, bring the upper arm forward and place it on the mat in front of the chest for support.

The foot of the upper leg is in the loop. The loop is in the arch of the foot with a tendency toward the heel. The upper leg is stretched upward in a slight outward rotation. <u>The foot is stretched.</u>

Purpose of the Exercise:

Stretch of the deep hip flexors and slight stretch of the leg backsides.
Mobilization of the hip joint.
Decoupling the leg movement from the hip and torso.
Slight strengthening of the inner thighs.

Execution: 5x - 10x per side

Pull the abdomen inward and upward. Stabilize the entire trunk with the muscles.

Image 2:	Stretch the upper leg forward as far as possible without otherwise changing the body position.
Image 3:	Stretch the leg upward vertically. This brings the leg into an outward rotation.
Image 4-5:	Now bring the upper leg as far backward and downward as possible without otherwise changing the body position and thereby falling into a hollow back.
Image 6:	Bring the leg back into the starting position,

Repeat 5x - 10x, then change the direction.

Image 7-8:	Pull the abdomen inward and upward and stretch the upper leg as far backward as possible without otherwise changing the body position and falling into a hollow back.
Image 9-10:	In a large circle, move the leg up into the vertical position. The leg is now rotated outward.
Image 11:	Stretch the upper leg as far forward and downward as possible without otherwise changing the body position. Do not round the back.
Image 12:	Bring the leg back into the starting position.

25. Ronde de Jambe (T)

4/4 Alternative name: Side Lying Big Leg Circles

Keep the pelvis as stable as possible, while, nonetheless, letting it react and naturally move into both directions. However, let neither the pelvis, nor the torso rotate forward or backward. Furthermore, there is no compression of the lumbar spine in the extension of the leg toward the hip or in the rounding with the leg flexed toward the hip. Therefore, particularly make sure to pull the abdominal muscles inward to protect the lower back.

Common Mistakes:

Viewed from above, there is no straight line. Usually, the torso and now sunk-in head are slightly tilted forward instead of remaining in one line with the leg on the mat.
The leg alternates in height on the way forward and backward.
The torso swings forward during the leg's backward and back-upward movement to compensate for the movement. The back is rounded during the leg's forward movement.
The leg is moved too far back during the backward movement, which causes a hollow back.
The back is rounded during the forward leg movement. The leg is moved too far back during the backward movement, which causes a hollow back.
The iliac spines (spina iliaca anterior superior) do not lie on top of each other, instead the upper edge of the pelvis is closer to the lowest rib.
The foot of the upper leg sickles (supination).
Within the circle there are positions in the movement that are less mobile. These are skipped.

Modifications or Variations:

For very tall people, the use of an additional carabiner can lengthen the leg springs so that the force at the end of the movement is not too great.
Keep the pelvis completely stable. This will reduce the radius of motion.
Instead of switching sides, continue with the one of the previous exercises.
Attach long, soft leg springs at a higher point on the Cadillac, if possible with Y-loops or gyro-double-loops that run both along the arch and around the ankle of the foot.
To make the exercise more difficult, bring the lower leg into one straight line with the rest of the body.

Contraindications/Risks:

Danger of luxation in case of fresh hip endoprostheses.

26. Magician Series Leg Circles (T)

1/3 Alternative name: Leg Springs Series in the air

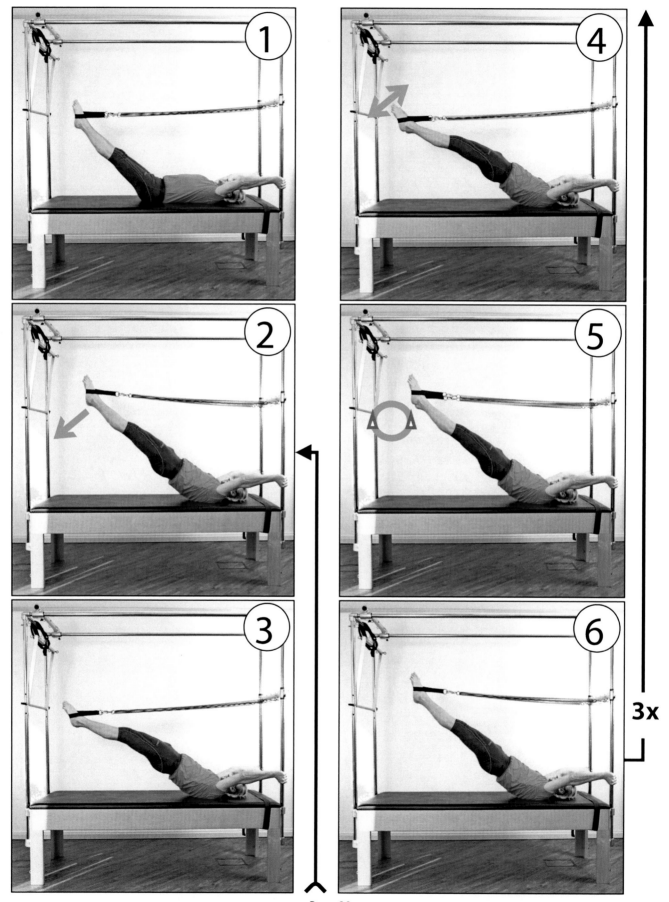

26. Magician Series Leg Circles (T)

2/3 Alternative name: Leg Springs Series in the air

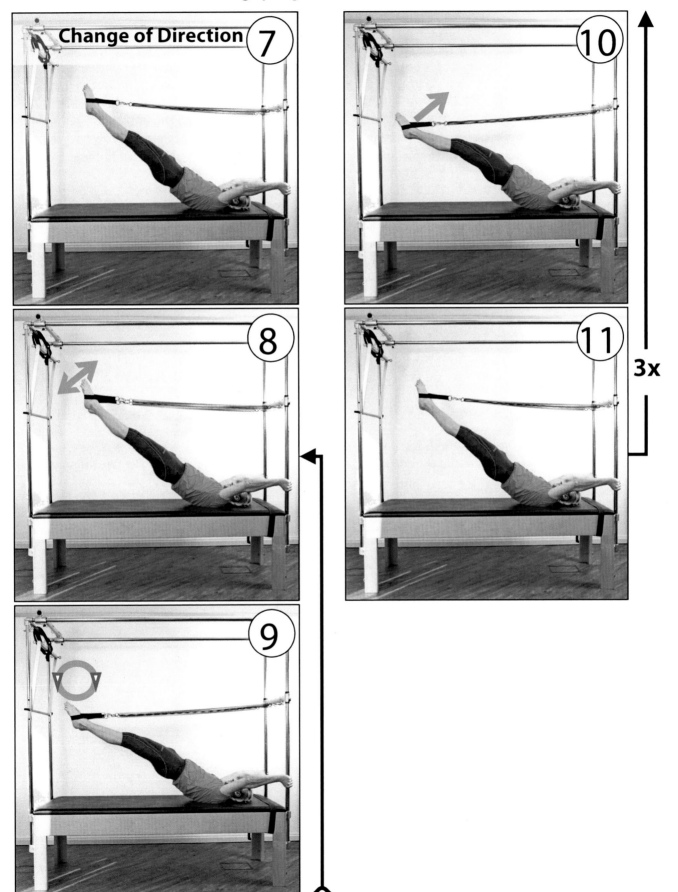

26. Magician Series Leg Circles (T)

3/3 Alternative name: Leg Springs Series up in the air

Setup:

Attach traditional leg springs at a height of 80 - 85 cm / 31.5 - 33.5 inches. The higher the spring attachment, the easier raising the body into the diagonal becomes.

Supine position with the head pointing toward the spring attachments. The distance to the vertical bars of the Cadillac should be between half an arm-length and one arm-length. The further away, the easier raising the body becomes. The hands hold the vertical bars slightly above the shoulders. The grip plays a central role in this exercise. If the fingers are closed, the strength to hold the body in the diagonal can easily be taken from the shoulder musculature. If the exercise is supposed to be carried primarily by the abdominal, back and gluteal musculature, then stretch the fingers.

Pelvis in a neutral position, spine in a natural position. Feet in the loops, the loops are in the arch of the foot, tendentially closer to the heels. The legs are in a slight outward rotation, <u>feet in a small V</u> (heels together, toes apart) and stretched. The legs are stretched upward to approx. 45 degrees.

Purpose of the Exercise:

Strengthening through isometric contraction of the abdominal, back and gluteal muscles as well as the latissimus dorsi and triceps brachii.

Execution: 3x - 5x per side

Image 2:   Pull the abdomen inward and upward. Build up inner thigh tension and tilt the pelvis posteriorly. Then roll up vertebra by vertebra until a straight line is reached from the shoulders to the feet. Keep the feet at one height.

Image 2-6:   **Down Circle:** Lower the closed legs as far as possible without changing the height or tilt of the pelvis. Then move the legs outward and upward in an up to mat-wide "D" and finally close the legs. At this point the body is back in a long, straight line.

Repeat 3-5x, then either return to the starting position before changing the direction, or change directions immediately.

Image 8-11:   **Up Circle:** From the starting position, move the legs slightly outward and then bring them downward in a large "D". At the end, close the legs and bring them back into the starting position.

Repeat 3-5x, then either continue directly with the next exercise, "26th Magician Series Beats", or roll down slowly, still leaving the feet at the same height.

Common Mistakes:

The starting position is considerably higher than 45 degrees.
The legs sink during the first roll-up.
No straight line from the shoulders to the feet is reached.

Modifications or Variations:

Try different heights.
Attach long, soft leg springs at a higher point on the Cadillac, if possible with Y-loops or gyro-double-loops that run both along the arch and around the ankle of the foot.

Contraindications/Risks:

Danger of luxation in case of fresh hip endoprostheses.
Depending on the spring attachments, this exercise places an increased strain on the shoulder and should therefore only be performed by people with healthy shoulders.
If there is a lack of inner thigh tension, the M. Piriformis may be overstrained with a corresponding Piriformis syndrome.

27. Magician Series Beats (T)

1/2 Alternative name: (instead of Magician Series) Leg Springs Series up in the air

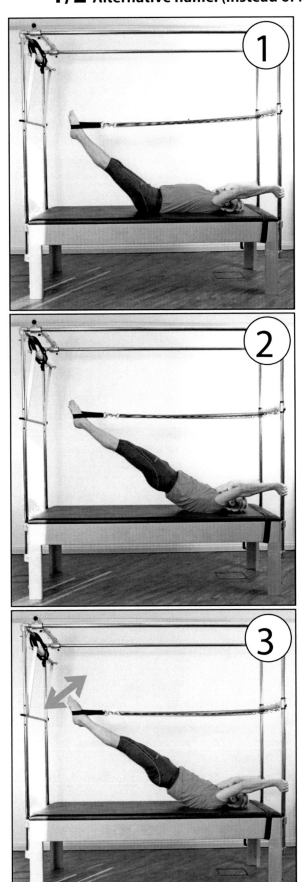

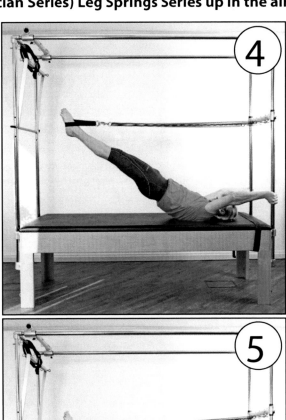

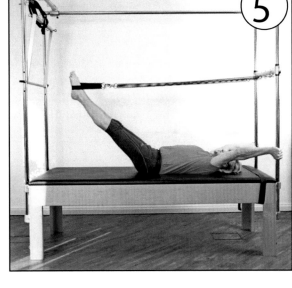

27. Magician Series Beats (T)

2/2 Alternative name: (instead of Magician Series) Leg Springs Series up in the air

Setup:

Attach traditional leg springs at a height of 80 - 85 cm / 31.5 - 33.5 inches. The higher the spring attachment, the easier raising the body into the diagonal becomes.

Supine position with the head pointing toward the spring attachments. The distance to the vertical bars of the Cadillac should be between half an arm-length and one arm-length. The further away, the easier raising the body becomes. The hands hold the vertical bars slightly above the shoulders. The grip plays a central role in this exercise. If the fingers are closed, the strength to hold the body in the diagonal can easily be taken from the shoulder musculature. If the exercise is supposed to be carried primarily by the abdominal, back and gluteal musculature, then stretch the fingers.

Pelvis in a neutral position, spine in a natural position. Feet in the loops, the loops are in the arch of the foot, tendentially closer to the heels. The legs are in a slight outward rotation, <u>feet in a small V</u> (heels together, toes apart) and stretched. The legs are stretched upward to approx. 45 degrees.

Purpose of the Exercise:

Strengthening through isometric contraction of the abdominal, back and gluteal muscles as well as the latissimus dorsi and triceps brachii.
Strengthening of the inner thighs.
Maintaining control over the springs.

Execution: 3x set with up to 10 repetitions

Image 2: Pull the abdomen inward and upward, build up inner thigh tension and tilt the pelvis posteriorly. Then roll up vertebra by vertebra until a straight line is reached from the shoulders to the feet. Keep the feet at the same height.

Image 3: Separate the heels slightly and then close them dynamically and quickly. Perform the entire exercise on one level.
10 repetitions. Pause.
10 repetitions. Pause.
10 repetitions.

Then either continue directly with the next exercise in the classic sequence, "29th Magician Series Bicycle", or roll down slowly while still keeping the feet at the same height.

Common Mistakes:

The starting position is considerably higher than 45 degrees.
The legs sink during the first roll-up.
No straight line from the shoulders to the feet is reached.
The springs begin to vibrate in one of their own natural frequencies, which can build up and become dangerous. Instead, keep the springs as steady as possible and counteract the proper motion of the springs.

Modifications or Variations:

Try different heights.
Attach long, soft leg springs at a higher point on the Cadillac, if possible with Y-loops or gyro-double-loops that run both along the arch and around the ankle of the foot.

Contraindications/Risks:

Depending on the spring attachments, this exercise places an increased strain on the shoulder and should therefore only be performed by people with healthy shoulders.
If there is a lack of inner thigh tension, the M. Piriformis may be overstrained with a corresponding Piriformis syndrome.

28. Magician Series Walking Prep (M)

1/2 Alternative name: (instead of Magician Series) Leg Springs Series up in the air

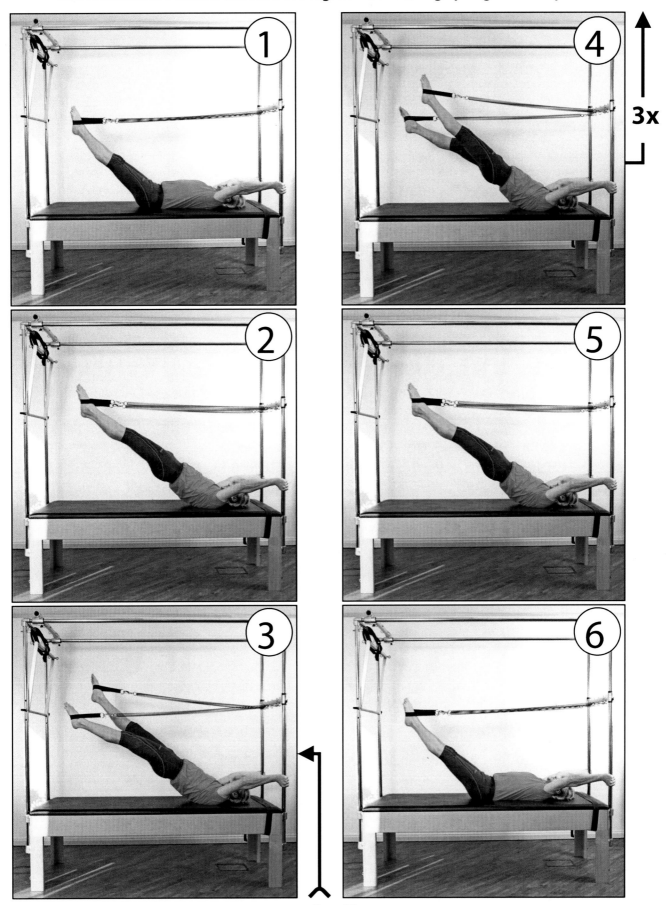

28. Magician Series Walking Prep (M)

2/2 Alternative name: (instead of Magician Series) Leg Springs Series up in the air

Setup:

Attach traditional leg springs at a height of 80 - 85 cm / 31.5 - 33.5 inches. The higher the spring attachment, the easier raising the body into the diagonal becomes.

Supine position with the head pointing toward the spring attachments. The distance to the vertical bars of the Cadillac should be between half an arm-length and one arm-length. The further away, the easier raising the body becomes. The hands hold the vertical bars slightly above the shoulders. The grip plays a central role in this exercise. If the fingers are closed, the strength to hold the body in the diagonal can easily be taken from the shoulder musculature. If the exercise is supposed to be carried primarily by the abdominal, back and gluteal musculature, then stretch the fingers.

Pelvis in a neutral position, spine in a natural position. Feet in the loops, the loops are in the arch of the foot, tendentially closer to the heels. The legs and <u>feet are parallel</u> and stretched. The legs are stretched upward to approx. 45 degrees.

Purpose of the Exercise:

Strengthening through isometric contraction of the abdominal, back and gluteal muscles as well as the latissimus dorsi and triceps brachii.
Strengthening of the inner thighs.

Execution: 1x set with 3 - 7 repetitions

Image 2: Pull the abdomen inward and upward, build up inner thigh tension and tilt the pelvis posteriorly. Then roll up vertebra by vertebra until a straight line is reached from the shoulders to the feet. Keep the feet at the same height.

Image 3: Slightly lower the left leg without changing the height and tilt of the pelvis. Raise the right leg slightly to the same extent.

Image 4: While the left leg moves up to the height of the right leg, lower the right leg.

Repeat 3-7x, the slowly roll down, keeping the feet at one height.

Common Mistakes:

The starting position is considerably higher than 45 degrees.
The legs are lowered during the first roll-up.
No straight line from the shoulders to the feet is reached.
The springs begin to vibrate in one of their own natural frequencies, which can build up and become dangerous. Instead, keep the springs as steady as possible and counteract the proper motion of the springs.

Modifications or Variations:

Try different heights.
Attach long, soft leg springs at a higher point on the Cadillac, if possible with Y-loops or gyro-double-loops that run both along the arch and around the ankle of the foot.

Contraindications/Risks:

Danger of luxation in case of fresh hip endoprostheses.
Depending on the spring attachments, this exercise places an increased strain on the shoulder and should therefore only be performed by people with healthy shoulders.
If there is a lack of inner thigh tension, the M. Piriformis may be overstrained with a corresponding Piriformis syndrome.

29. Magician Series Walking (T)

1/4 Alternative name: (instead of Magician Series) Leg Springs Series up in the air

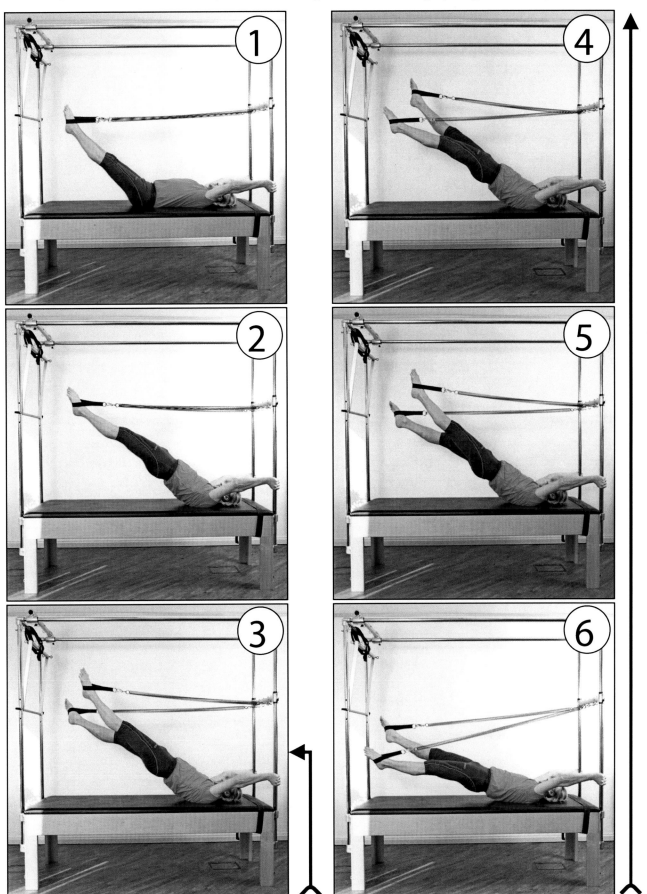

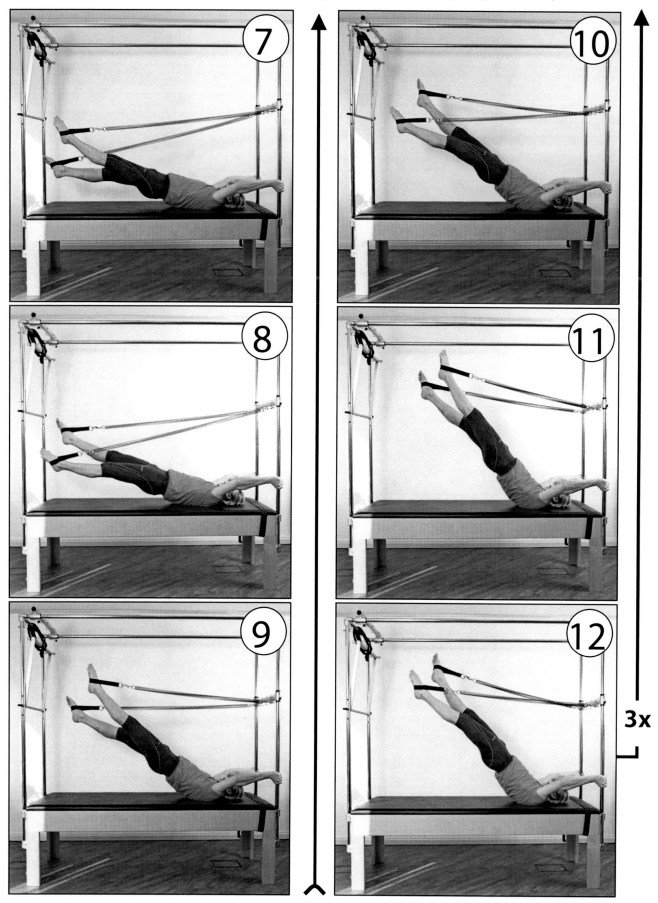

3x

29. Magician Series Walking (T)

3/4 Alternative name: (instead of Magician Series) Leg Springs Series up in the air

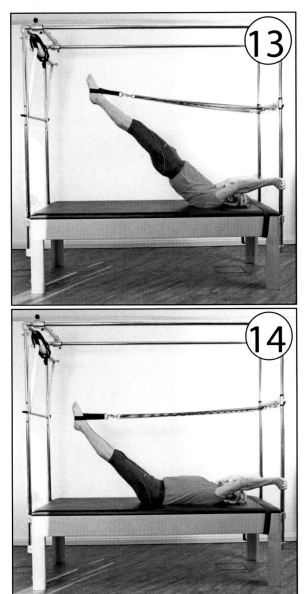

29. Magician Series Walking (T)

4/4 Alternative name: (instead of Magician Series) Leg Springs Series up in the air

Setup:

Attach traditional leg springs at a height of 80 - 85 cm / 31.5 - 33.5 inches. The higher the spring attachment, the easier raising the body into the diagonal becomes.

Supine position with the head pointing toward the spring attachments. The distance to the vertical bars of the Cadillac should be between half an arm-length and one arm-length. The further away, the easier raising the body becomes. The hands hold the vertical bars slightly above the shoulders. The grip plays a central role in this exercise. If the fingers are closed, the strength to hold the body in the diagonal can easily be taken from the shoulder musculature. If the exercise is supposed to be carried primarily by the abdominal, back and gluteal musculature, then stretch the fingers.

Pelvis in a neutral position, spine in a natural position. Feet in the loops, the loops are in the arch of the foot, tendentially closer to the heels. The legs and <u>feet are parallel</u> and stretched. The legs are stretched upward to approx. 45 degrees.

Purpose of the Exercise:

Strengthening through isometric contraction of the abdominal, back and gluteal muscles as well as the latissimus dorsi and triceps brachii.
Strengthening of the inner thighs.

Execution: 3 - 5 repetitions

Image 2:   Pull the abdomen inward and upward, build up inner thigh tension and tilt the pelvis posteriorly. Then roll up vertebra by vertebra until a straight line from the shoulders to the feet is reached. Keep the feet at the same height.

Image 3:   Slightly lower the left leg without changing the height and tilt of the pelvis. Raise the right leg slightly to the same extent.

Image 4:   While the left leg moves up to the height of the right leg, lower the right leg.

Image 5-12:   As the legs move in opposite directions, the body moves even further upward in a straight line. Be careful not to strain the cervical spine. Continue the leg movement, lowering the whole body in a long line as far down as possible and, finally, coming back up.

Repeat this pending up and down movement 3-5x, then come back into the starting position and roll down slowly, still keeping the feet at the same height.

Common Mistakes:

The starting position is considerably higher than 45 degrees.
The legs sink during the first roll-up.
No straight line from the shoulders to the feet is reached.
The springs begin to vibrate in one of their own natural frequencies, which can build up and become dangerous. Instead, keep the springs as steady as possible and counteract the proper motion of the springs.

Modifications or Variations:

Attach long, soft leg springs at a higher point on the Cadillac, if possible with Y-loops or gyro-double-loops that run both along the arch and around the ankle of the foot.

Contraindications/Risks:

Danger of luxation in case of fresh hip endoprostheses.
This exercise places an increased strain on the shoulder and should therefore only be performed by people with healthy shoulders.
If there is a lack of inner thigh tension, the M. Piriformis may be overstrained with a corresponding Piriformis syndrome.

30. Magician Series Bicycle (T)

1/4 Alternative name: (instead of Magician Series) Leg Springs Series up in the air

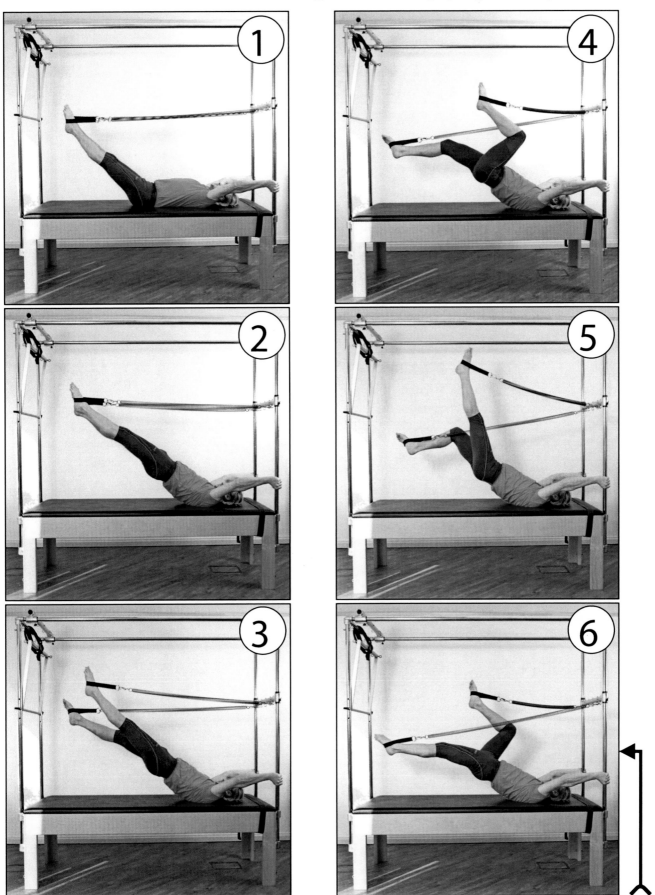

30. Magician Series Bicycle (T)

2/4 Alternative name: (instead of Magician Series) Leg Springs Series up in the air

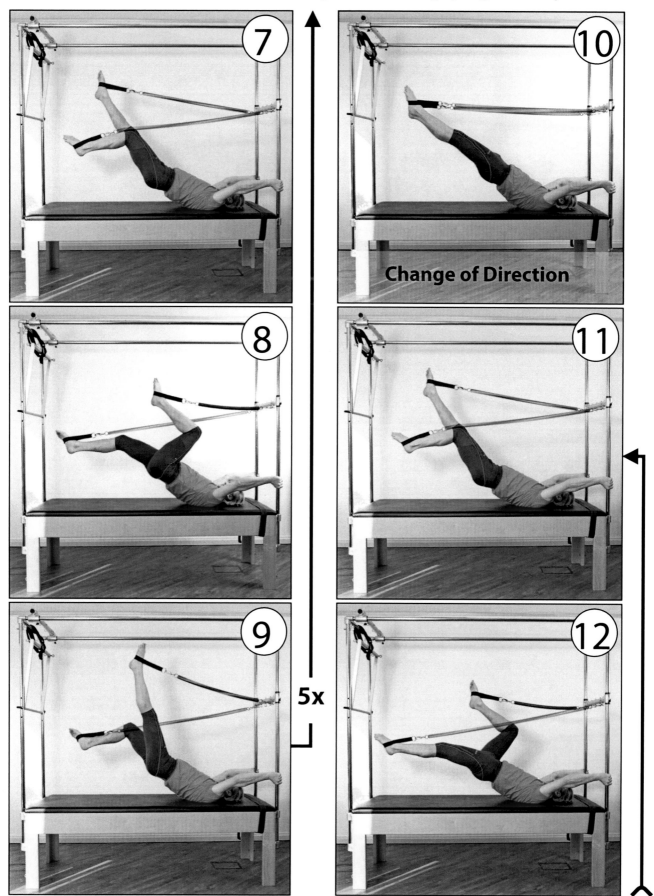

Change of Direction

5x

30. Magician Series Bicycle (T)

3/4 Alternative name: (instead of Magician Series) Leg Springs Series up in the air

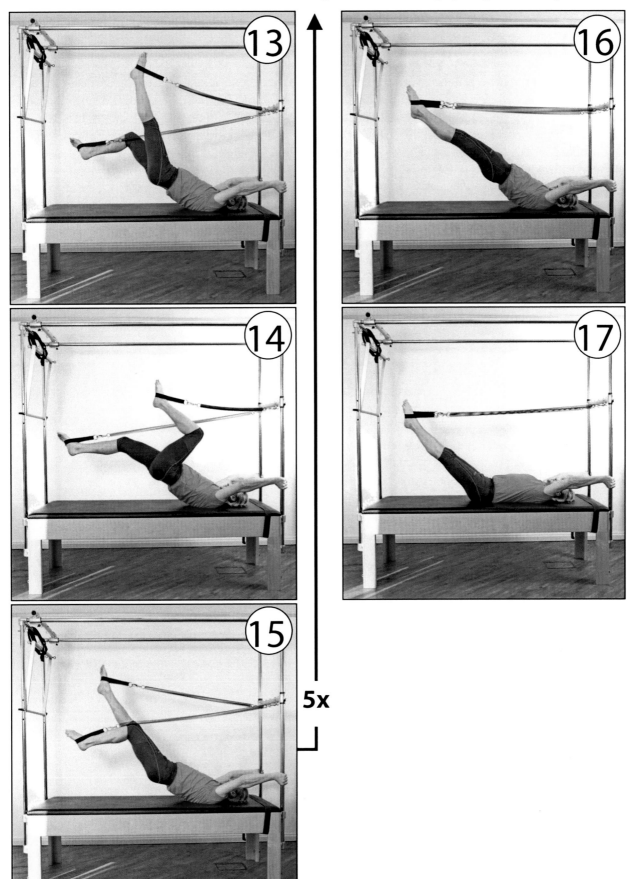

30. Magician Series Bicycle (T)

4/4 Alternative name: (instead of Magician Series) Leg Springs Series up in the air

Setup:

Attach traditional leg springs at a height of 80 - 85 cm / 31.5 - 33.5 inches. The higher the spring attachment, the easier raising the body into the diagonal becomes.

Supine position with the head pointing toward the spring attachments. The distance to the vertical bars of the Cadillac should be between half an arm-length and one arm-length. The further away, the easier raising the body becomes. The hands hold the vertical bars slightly above the shoulders. The grip plays a central role in this exercise. If the fingers are closed, the strength to hold the body in the diagonal can easily be taken from the shoulder musculature. If the exercise is supposed to be carried primarily by the abdominal, back and gluteal musculature, then stretch the fingers.

Pelvis in a neutral position, spine in a natural position. Feet in the loops, the loops are in the arch of the foot, tendentially closer to the heels. The legs and <u>feet are parallel</u> and stretched. The legs are stretched upward to approx. 45 degrees.

Purpose of the Exercise:

Strengthening through isometric contraction of the abdominal, back and gluteal muscles as well as the latissimus dorsi and triceps brachii.
Strengthening of the inner thighs.

Execution: 5x - 7x repetitions

Image 2: Pull the abdomen inward and upward, build up inner thigh tension and tilt the pelvis posteriorly. Then roll up vertebra by vertebra until a straight line from the shoulders to the feet is reached. Keep the feet at the same height.

Image 3: Slightly lower the right stretched leg and slightly raise the left stretched leg.

Image 4-5: Bend the left leg, pull it toward the chest and then stretch it upward and forward. Simultaneously, lower the right leg even further and then bend it.

Image 6-7: Bend the right leg, pull it toward the chest and then stretch it upward and forward. Simultaneously, lower the left leg even further and then bend it.

Image 8-9: Bend the left leg, pull it toward the chest and then stretch it upward and forward. Simultaneously, lower the right leg even further and then bend it.

Repeat the sequence from image 6 to 9 for 5-7x , then change the direction or roll down for a pause.

Common Mistakes:

The starting position is considerably higher than 45 degrees.
The legs sink during the first roll-up.
No straight line from the shoulders to the feet is reached.
The leg movement is not harmonious and round. For example, one of the knees always slides outward.

Modifications or Variations:

Try different heights.
Attach long, soft leg springs at a higher point on the Cadillac, if possible with Y-loops or gyro-double-loops that run both along the arch and around the ankle of the foot.

Contraindications/Risks:

Danger of luxation in case of fresh hip endoprostheses.
This exercise places an increased strain on the shoulder and should therefore only be performed by people with healthy shoulders.
If there is a lack of inner thigh tension, the M. Piriformis may be overstrained with a corresponding Piriformis syndrome.

31. Airplane (T)

1/4 Alternative name: part of the Magician Series

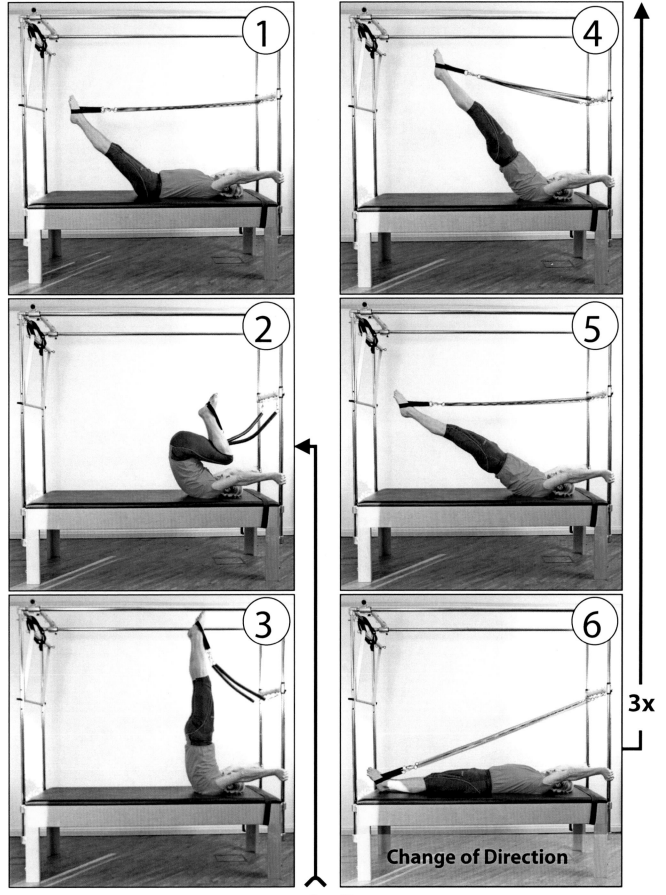

Change of Direction

3x

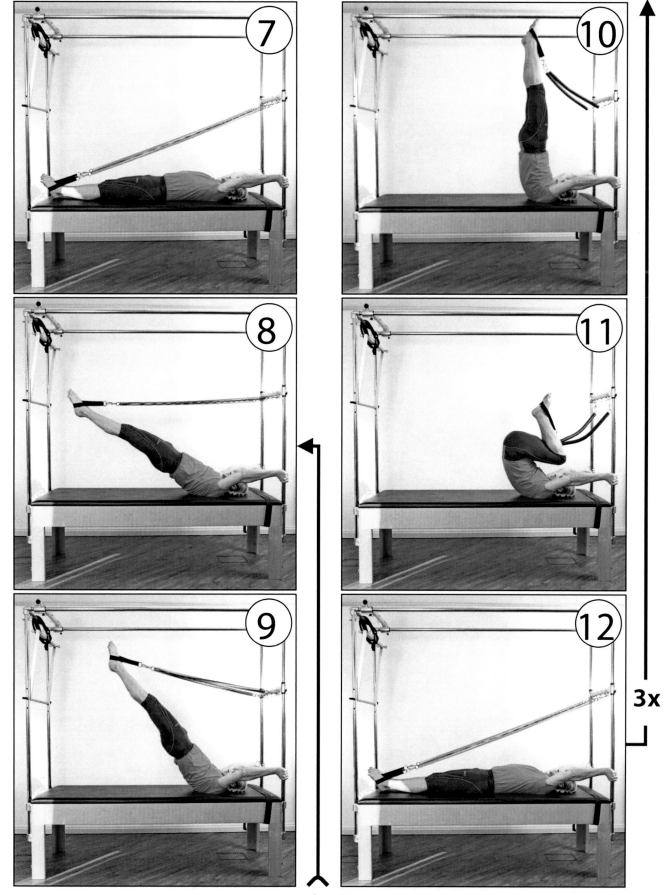

31. Airplane (T)

3/4 Alternative name: part of the Magician Series

Setup:

Attach traditional leg springs at a height of 80 - 85 cm / 31.5 - 33.5 inches. The higher the spring attachment, the easier raising the body into the diagonal becomes.

Supine position with the head pointing toward the spring attachments. The distance to the vertical bars of the Cadillac should be between half an arm-length and one arm-length. The further away, the easier raising the body becomes. The hands hold the vertical bars slightly above the shoulders. The grip plays a central role in this exercise. If the fingers are closed, the strength to hold the body in the diagonal can easily be taken from the shoulder musculature. If the exercise is supposed to be carried primarily by the abdominal, back and gluteal musculature, then stretch the fingers.

Pelvis in a neutral position, spine in a natural position. Feet in the loops, the loops are in the arch of the foot, tendentially closer to the heels. The legs are in a slight outward rotation, <u>feet in a small V</u> (heels together, toes apart) and stretched. The legs are raised to approx. 45 degrees.

Purpose of the Exercise:

Strengthening of the shoulder, abdominal, back and gluteal muscles.
Strengthening of the inner thighs.
Mobilization of the spine.

Execution: 3x - 5x repetitions

Image 2: Pull the abdomen inward and upward, build up inner thigh tension and tilt the pelvis posteriorly. Simultaneously, pull the knees to the chest and roll up vertebrae by vertebra until, normally, the knees are above the eyes.

Image 3: Now stretch the legs upward and form a straight and vertical line with the body. The springs are mostly relaxed in this position. Make sure that the neck is not under pressure. Correct the body line according to the ideal of the vertical until a strain-free position is reached. For further repetitions directly strive for this angle.

Image 4-6: With the body stretched and the shoulders as the axis, move the legs away from the spring attachments. At one point the springs begin to stretch and thereby support the "landing procedure". Lower the legs and roll down slowly until the end of the mat is reached.

Then bend the legs again and repeat the sequence from image 2 to 6 for 3-5x, then change the direction.

Image 7-10: Pull the abdomen inward and upward and build up inner thigh tension. Slowly raise the stretched body until the vertical or individually suitable position for the body is reached. Again, the shoulder belt is the axis of movement.

Image 11-12: Now, bend the knees and bring them above the eyes. Hold this position and slowly roll down vertebra by vertebra as a "ball" until the pelvis is back in its neutral position. Now stretch the legs out on the Cadillac mat. Different from the exercise on the Reformer, the springs do not support the roll-down here. Hence, come down in a particularly controlled manner.

Repeat the sequence from image 8 to 12 for 3-5x.

31. Airplane (T)

4/4 Alternative name: part of the Magician Series

Common Mistakes:

During the stretched lowering, the body falls into the springs and from there, sinks down relatively uncontrolled.

After the change of direction the body comes up too fast and the springs slam shut.

The unsupported part of the roll-down is performed too quickly.

Modifications or Variations:

Try different spring attachment heights.

Attach long, soft leg springs at a higher point on the Cadillac, if possible with Y-loops or gyro-double-loops that run both along the arch and around the ankle of the foot.

A variation that can be performed with both spring types is exercise " 31. Flying Airplane Variation".

Perform the first direction without springs. Ideally, slide so close to the vertical bars of the Cadillac that the angle of the arms is very small. Alternatively, if possible, hold the edge of the Cadillac mat over the head (elbows and palms pointing upward).

Contraindications/Risks:

This exercise places an increased strain on the shoulder and should therefore only be performed by people with healthy shoulders.

If there is a lack of inner thigh tension, the M. Piriformis may be overstrained with a corresponding Piriformis syndrome.

32. Flying Airplane Variation (M)
1/4

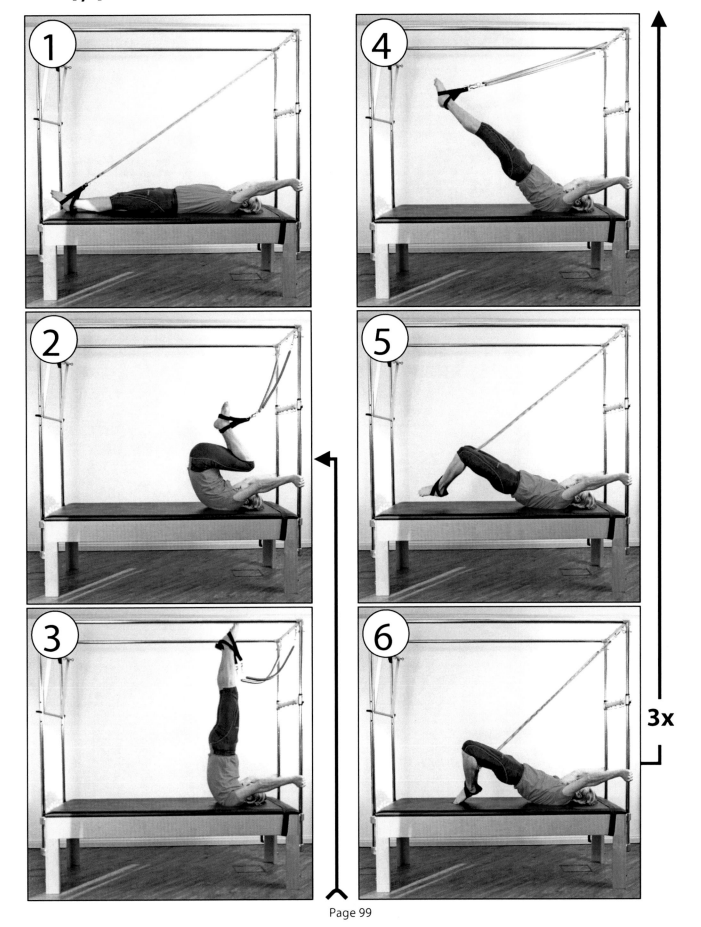

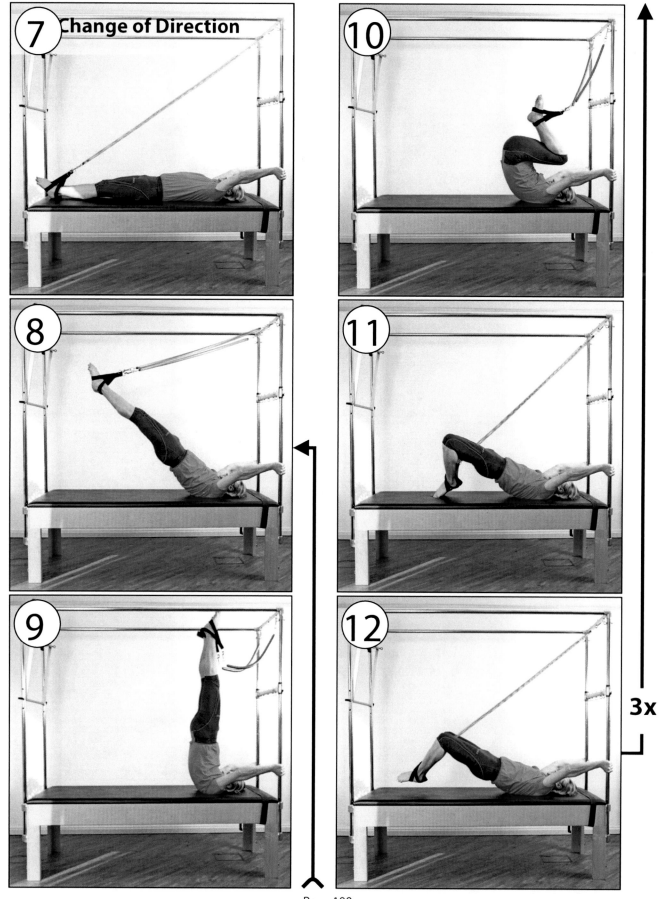

32. Flying Airplane Variation (M)
3/4

Setup:

Select the spring position so that the exercise can be performed completely and without any evasive movements. The height of the spring position also influences the effect of the exercise. Typically, the long, soft leg springs are attached at the highest possible point of the Cadillac. Ideally, use Y-loops or gyro-double-loops that run both along the arch and around the ankle of the foot.

Supine position with the head pointing toward the spring attachments. The distance to the vertical bars of the Cadillac should be between half an arm-length and one arm-length. The further away, the easier raising the body becomes. The hands hold the vertical bars slightly above the shoulders. The grip plays a central role in this exercise. If the fingers are closed, the strength to hold the body in the diagonal can easily be taken from the shoulder musculature. If the exercise is supposed to be carried primarily by the abdominal, back and gluteal musculature, then stretch the fingers.

Pelvis in a neutral position, spine in a natural position. Feet in the loops, the loops are in the arch of the foot, tendentially closer to the heels. The legs are in a slight outward rotation, <u>feet in a small V</u> (heels together, toes apart) and stretched. The legs are stretched out on the Cadillac mat.

Purpose of the Exercise:

Strengthening of the shoulder, abdominal, back and gluteal muscles.
Mobilization of the spine.

Execution: 3x - 5x repetitions

Image 2: Pull the abdomen inward and upward, build up inner thigh tension and bend the knees, pulling them toward the head. As soon as the knees are above the pelvis, tilt the pelvis posteriorly. Simultaneously, pull the knees to the chest and roll up vertebrae by vertebra until, normally, the knees are above the eyes.

Image 3: Now stretch the legs upward and form a straight and vertical line with the body. The springs are mostly relaxed in this position. Make sure that the neck is not under pressure. Correct the body line according to the ideal of the vertical until a strain-free position is reached. For further repetitions directly strive for this angle.

Image 4: With the body stretched and the shoulders as the axis, move away from the spring attachments. At one point the springs begin to stretch and thereby support the "landing procedure". Lower the legs until the end of the mat is reached.

Image 5-6: Bend the knees and open them slightly. The rest of the body remains at the previous height. Now drag the toes across the Cadillac mat with light contact. Then pull the knees toward the chest and come directly into the position of image 2.

Then bend the legs again and repeat the sequence from image 2 to 6 for 3-5x.

Image 7: Lie on the Cadillac with the body stretched out. Pull the abdomen inward and upward and build up inner thigh tension.

Image 8-9: Pull the abdomen inward and upward and build up inner thigh tension. Slowly raise the stretched body until the vertical or individually suitable position for the body is reached. Again, the shoulder belt is the axis of movement.

Image 10-11: Now, bend the knees and bring them above the eyes. Instead of the complete roll-down, perform something like a "high jumping" movement as in exercise "26. Rolling in and out" with the Roll-Down Bar (Cadillac Manual Part 1). The toes lightly touch the Cadillac mat.

Image 12: Keep the hip at the reached height and slowly stretch the legs. Push forward on the Cadillac mat with the toes for as long as possible until they loose contact to the mat and the legs are fully stretched.

Repeat the sequence from image 8 to 12 for 3-5x.

32. Flying Airplane Variation (M)
4/4

Common Mistakes:

The pelvis does not hold the height in image 5-6 and image 11-12, and/or the feet push too hard into the mat and therefore hold part of the weight.

Modifications or Variations:

Attach traditional leg springs at a height of 80 - 85 cm / 31.5 - 33.5 inches.

Contraindications/Risks:

This exercise places an increased strain on the shoulder and should therefore only be performed by people with healthy shoulders.

If there is a lack of inner thigh tension, the M. Piriformis may be overstrained with a corresponding Piriformis syndrome.

33. Coordination (T)
1/2

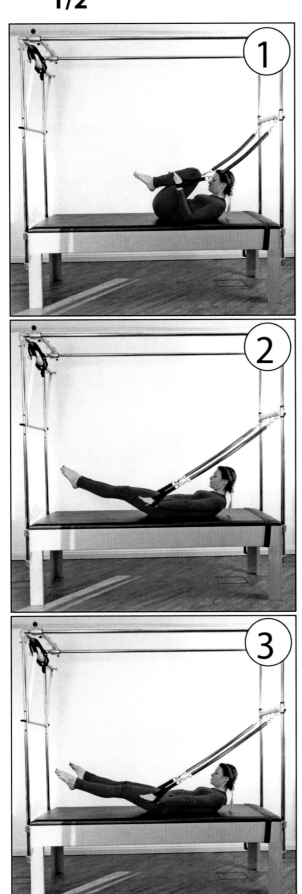

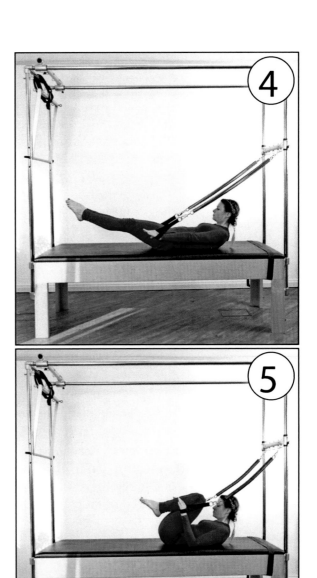

33. Coordination (T)
2/2

Setup:

Attach traditional leg springs at a height of 80 - 85 cm / 31.5 - 33.5 inches.
Supine position with the head pointing toward the spring attachments. The head lies at the end of the Cadillac mat or with some distance away from it. The further away, the harder stretching the arms and raising the upper body becomes. The hands are either in the loops or they hold the loops like ropes.
The knees are slightly opened and pulled toward the chest, which brings the pelvis into a slight posterior tilt and makes the lumbar spine flatten a bit. Feet in a small V (heels together, toes apart) and stretched. Bend the elbows and bring them close to the body. The springs are not stretched yet. The head and chest are raised slightly. The tips of the scapulae are barely still touching the Cadillac mat.

Purpose of the Exercise:

Strengthening of the vertical abdominal muscles, the deep hip flexors, the triceps under the control of the arm adductors (M. triceps brachii (caput longum), M. latissimus dorsi, M. pectoralis major, M. teres major, M. teres minor, M. coracobrachialis).
Breathing exercise.

Execution: 5x - 7x

Image 2: Exhaling steadily, stretch the arms out on / slightly above the Cadillac mat and close to the body. Still exhaling, stretch the legs shortly after the arms initiated the movement. The idea is that "the arms stretch the legs". The legs remain in the outward rotation. The height of the legs above the mat depends on the individual abilities of the person performing the exercise. The lowest position that can gradually be achieved is on eye-level.

Image 3-4: Holding the breath, open the legs and close them again.

Image 5: Breathing in steadily, bend the legs and pull them toward the head. Shortly after starting this movement, bend the elbows. The idea is that "the legs bring the arms back".

Common Mistakes:

Danger of a hollow back, make sure to raise the legs high enough.
The upper body is gradually lowered during the exercise.
Instead of rolling up with the chest and keeping the head relatively vertical, the lacking flexion of the upper body is reached by over-flexing the head. This can often be seen through the chin almost lying on the chest. In this position, the muscles of the front of the throat are overstrained and the airways are partly blocked.
The head is pushed too far forward, causing an overstraining of the sternocleidomastoid. This can be felt at the tip behind the ears.
The arms are not fully stretched.
The shoulders wing, causing an over-accentuation of the pectoralis.
The wrists are not sufficiently stabilized and therefore unnecessarily dorsally extended.

Modifications or Variations:

Perform the exercise without lifting the head.

Contraindications/Risks:

In case of preexisting problems with the cervical spine, the continuous flexion can worsen the problem.
Danger of an overstraining of the lumbar spine if the spine cannot be held down on the mat.

34. Flying Eagle (T)
1/3

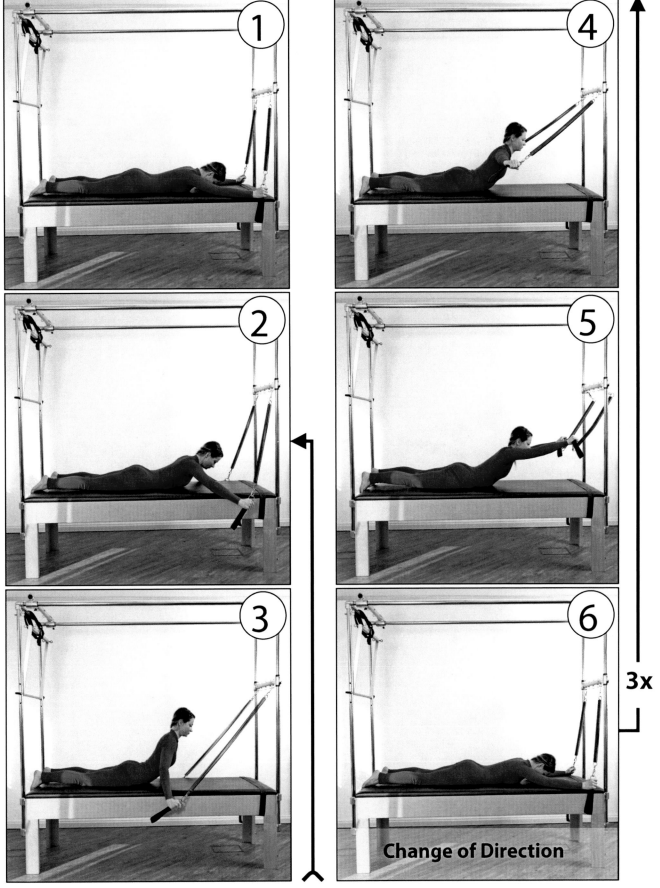

1

2

3

4

5

6

Change of Direction

3x

34. Flying Eagle (T)
2/3

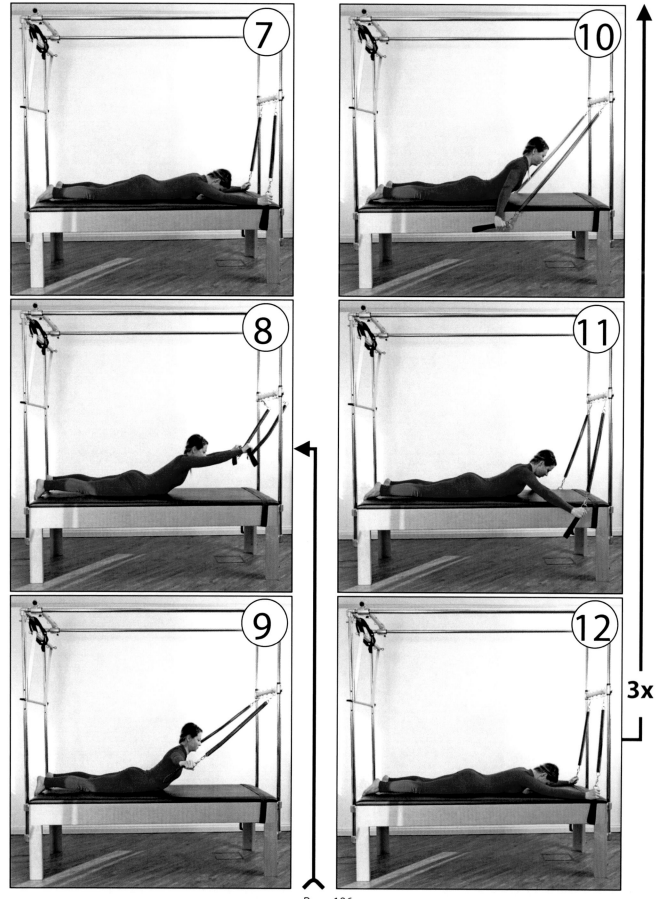

34. Flying Eagle (T)
3/3

Setup:

Attach traditional leg springs at a height of 80 - 85 cm / 31.5 - 33.5 inches.
Prone position, one arm-length away from the vertical bars of the Cadillac.
The hands hold the loops like ropes. Ideally, the fingertips press the loops into the balls of the thumb. The arms are stretched out to the right and left side of the Cadillac mat.
The head is slightly lifted, looking down, so that the nose does not touch the mat. Ideally, the legs are closed, or alternatively opened so far that the lower back is comfortable during the exercise.
Conversely, closing the legs can reduce the amount of work done by the lower back muscles. If the body height allows it, reach around the back edge of the Cadillac with the toes.

Purpose of the Exercise:

Strengthening of the entire back musculature, the latissimus dorsi, triceps and the posterior part of the deltoid.
If the feet can reach around the Cadillac end, there is a strengthening of the foot lifters.
Improvement of the extension capacity of the spine.

Execution: 3x - 6x per direction

Image 2-3: Pull the abdomen inward to distribute the strain on the spine as evenly as possible. Raise the head and chest and come up as high as possible. Simultaneously, pull the leg springs down past the Cadillac and then as far backward as possible, into the direction of the outer leg sides.
Image 4-5: Maintain the reached height of the chest as much as possible and move the springs outward and forward in a large curve.
Image 6: Lower the upper body again.
Repeat 3x - 5x, then change the direction.

Image 7-8: Maintain the reached height of the chest as much as possible and move the springs outward and forward in a large curve. Simultaneously, raise the arms.
Image 9: Maintain the reached height of the chest as much as possible and move the springs backward, into the direction of the outer leg sides, in a large curve.
Image 10-11: Move the arms downward and forward along the sides of the Cadillac. Keep the upper body raised as high as possible.
Image 12: Lower the upper body again.
Repeat 3x - 5x.

Common Mistakes:

The head is overstretched too strongly to conceal the lacking flexibility of the thoracic spine.
The movement is performed too much by the lumbar spine.

Modifications or Variations:

Instead of performing a circular movement, move the arms backward and then back to the front, similar to the Reformer exercise "Pulling Straps 1".
Perform the exercise while lying on a Reformer-Box. Accordingly, attach the springs at a higher point.
Use soft springs with less "uplift".

Contraindications/Risks:

Back problems, which make extensions painful.
Shoulder problems.

35. Backstroke (T)
1/3

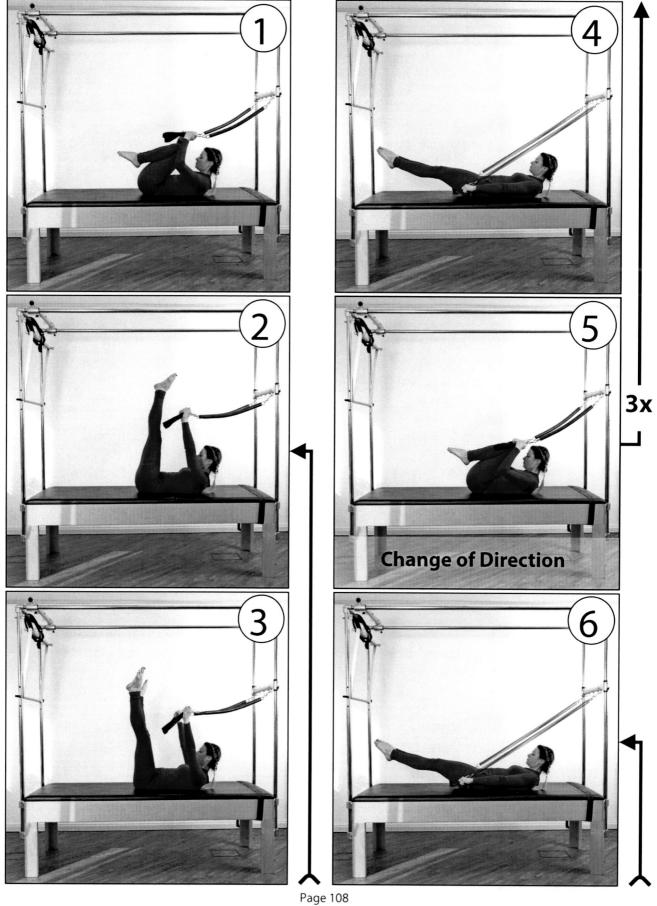

Change of Direction

3x

35. Backstroke (T)
2/3

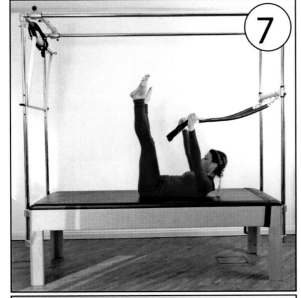

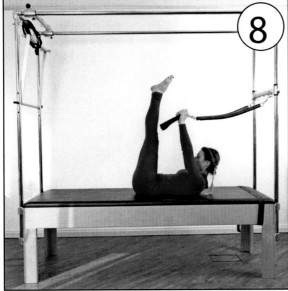

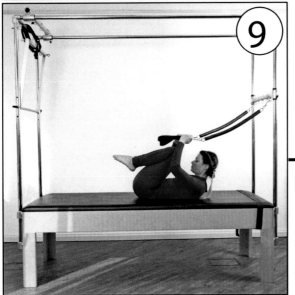

3x

Setup:

Attach traditional leg springs at a height of 80 - 85 cm / 31.5 - 33.5 inches.

Supine position with the head pointing toward the spring attachments. The head lies at the end of the Cadillac mat or with some distance away from it. The further away, the harder stretching the arms and raising the upper body becomes. The hands hold the loops like ropes.

The knees are slightly opened and pulled toward the chest, which brings the pelvis into a slight posterior tilt and makes the lumbar spine flatten a bit. <u>Feet in a small V</u> (heels together, toes apart) and stretched. The elbows are bent to the sides, the fists press against each other. The springs are not stretched yet. The head and chest are raised slightly. The tips of the scapulae are barely still touching the Cadillac mat.

Purpose of the Exercise:

Strengthening of the vertical abdominal muscles, the hip flexors, and the latissimus dorsi.

35. Backstroke (T)
3/3

Execution: 5x - 7x

Image 2: Stretch the arms and legs upward almost parallel to each other. The legs are closed and the arms shoulder-wide apart.

Image 3: The legs and arms open approx. to the width of the Cadillac.

Image 4: Bring the legs and arms forward in a parabolic curve. Close the legs and press the stretched arms against the sides of the body. The legs remain in the outward rotation. The height of the legs above the mat depends on the individual abilities of the person performing the exercise. The lowest position that can gradually be achieved, according to Joseph Pilates' instructions for comparable mat exercises, is at approx. 5 cm / 2 inches. Hold for a short moment and try to roll up slightly further without changing the position of the legs.

Image 5: Come back into the starting position without lowering the upper body or head.

Repeat 3x - 5x, then change the direction.

Image 6: Bring the legs and arms forward. The legs are closed, stretched out and slightly rotated outward with the feet in a small V. The stretched arms press against the sides of the body. The height of the legs above the mat depends on the individual abilities of the person performing the exercise. The lowest position that can gradually be achieved, according to Joseph Pilates' instructions for comparable mat exercises, is at approx. 5cm/2 inches.

Image 7: The legs and arms open approx. to the width of the Cadillac and move upward vertically.

Image 8: Close the legs and move the arms to shoulder-width.

Image 9: Come back into the starting position without lowering the upper body or head.

Repeat 3x - 5x.

Common Mistakes:

Danger of a hollow back, make sure to raise the legs high enough.
The upper body is gradually lowered during the exercise.
Instead of rolling up with the chest and keeping the head relatively vertical, the lacking flexion of the upper body is reached by over-flexing the head. The head is pushed too far forward, causing an overstraining of the sternocleidomastoid.
The arms are not fully stretched.
The shoulders wing, causing an over-accentuation of the pectoralis.
The wrists are not sufficiently stabilized and therefore unnecessarily dorsally extended.

Modifications or Variations:

Attach traditional leg springs at mat height.

Contraindications/Risks:

In case of preexisting problems with the cervical spine, the continuous flexion can worsen the problem.
Danger of an overstraining of the lumbar spine if the spine cannot be held down on the mat.

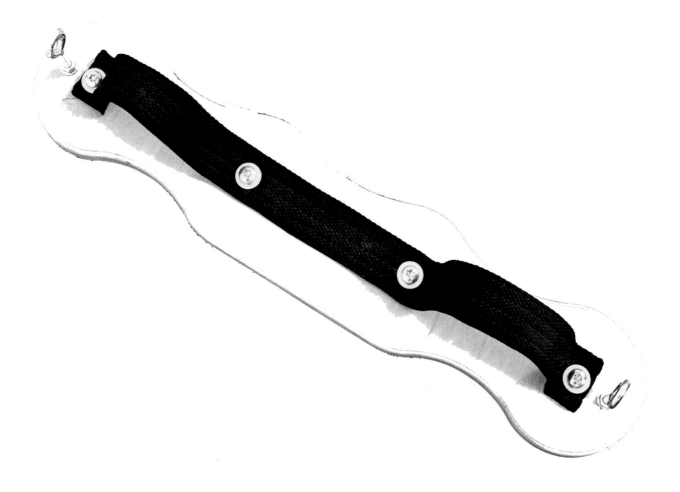

Airplane Board

Preliminary Remarks for the Airplane Board

The Airplane Board was developed by Joseph Pilates and can be seen on various film and archive photographs, e.g. on the 1951 LIFE Magazine photos where Joseph Pilates instructs Roberta Peters using the Airplane Board.

The Airplane Board is an assistance tool, which turns the unilateral exercises of the leg springs into bilateral exercises.

Compared to the loops of the leg springs, the Airplane Board offers more support. In addition, the chain between the legs is closed, which makes exercises, such as the Airplane series, much easier.

1. Airplane with Airplane Board (T)
1/4

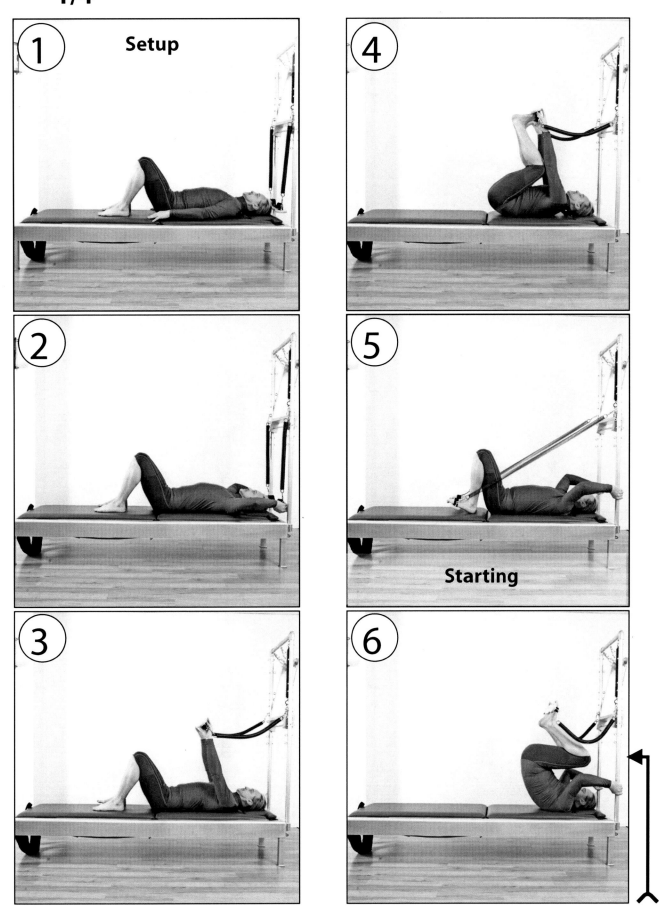

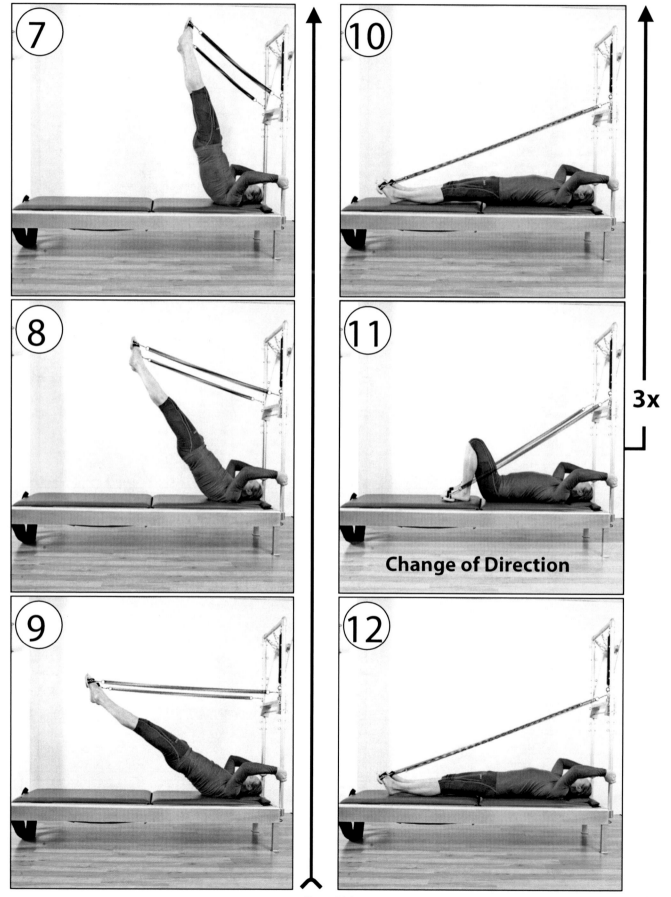

Change of Direction

3x

1. Airplane with Airplane Board (T)
3/4

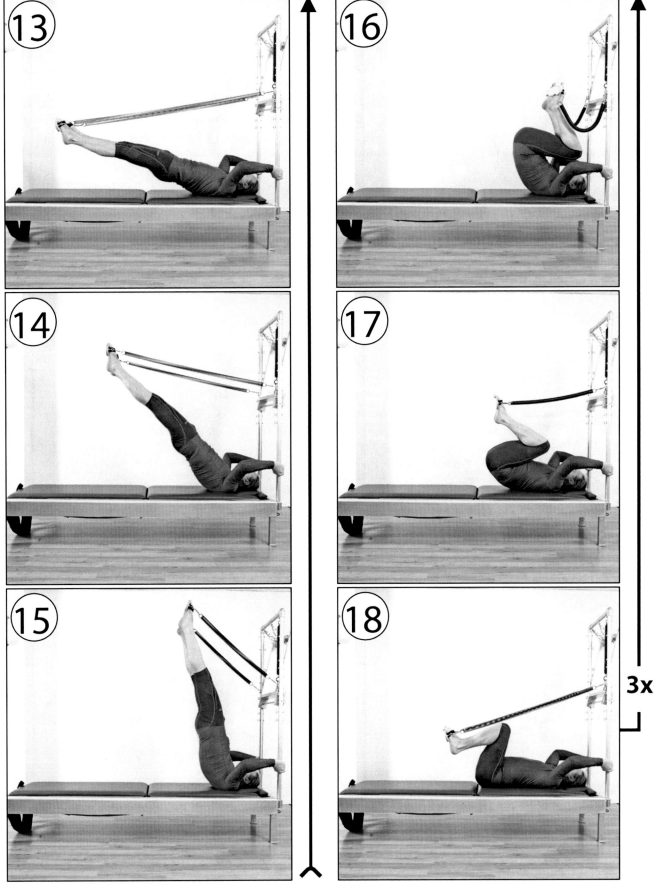

1. Airplane with Airplane Board (T)
4/4

Setup:

Attach traditional leg springs with the Airplane Board at a height of 80 - 85 cm / 31.5 - 33.5 inches. The higher the spring attachment, the more the leg backsides have to work.

Supine position with the head pointing toward the spring attachments. The distance to the vertical bars of the Cadillac should be between half an arm-length and one arm-length. The further away, the harder the exercise. The hands hold the Airplane Board. Securely place the feet in the Airplane Board. The hands hold the vertical bars slightly above the shoulders. Pelvis in a neutral position, spine in a natural position. The feet are behind the buttocks, the knees are bent. To have even more security with the feet in the board, press into the loops even more firmly when the legs are bent and the Airplane Board is fixed onto the mat.

Purpose of the Exercise:

Strengthening of the shoulder, abdominal, back and gluteal muscles.

Execution: 3x - 5x repetitions

Image 6:   Pull the abdomen inward and upward, build up inner thigh tension and tilt the pelvis posteriorly. Simultaneously, pull the knees to the chest and roll up vertebrae by vertebra until, normally, the knees are above the eyes.

Image 7:   Now stretch the legs upward and form a straight and vertical line with the body. The springs are mostly relaxed in this position. Make sure that the neck is not under pressure. Correct the body line according to the ideal of the vertical until a strain-free position is reached. For further repetitions directly strive for this angle.

Image 8-10: With the body stretched and the shoulders as the axis, move away from the spring attachments. At one point the springs begin to stretch and thereby support the "landing procedure". Come down stretched out until the body is completely laid down on the mat.

Image 11:   Bend the legs and bring the feet behind the buttocks.

Repeat the sequence from image 6 to 11 3-5x, then change the direction.

Image 12:   Stretch the legs out on the Cadillac mat until the body is completely laid down on the mat.

Image 13-15: Pull the abdomen inward and upward and build up inner thigh tension. Slowly raise the stretched body until the vertical or individually suitable position for the body is reached. Again, the shoulder belt is the axis of movement.

Image 16-18: Now, bend the knees and bring them above the eyes. Hold this position and slowly roll down vertebra by vertebra as a "ball" until the pelvis is back in its neutral position. Different from the Short Spine exercise on the Reformer, the springs do not support the roll down here. Hence, roll down in a particularly controlled manner.

Repeat the sequence from image 12 to 18 3-5x.

Common Mistakes:

During the stretched lowering, the body falls into the springs and from there, sinks down in a relatively uncontrolled manner.

After the change of direction the body comes up too fast and the springs slam shut.

The unsupported part of the roll-down is performed too quickly.

Modifications or Variations: -

Contraindications/Risks:

This exercise places an increased strain on the shoulder and should therefore only be performed by people with healthy shoulders.

2. Pressing out & Pulling in (T)

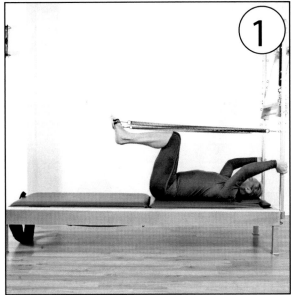

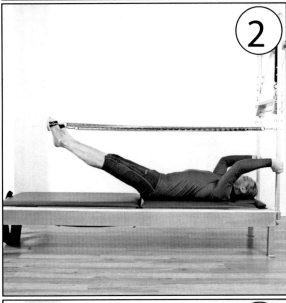

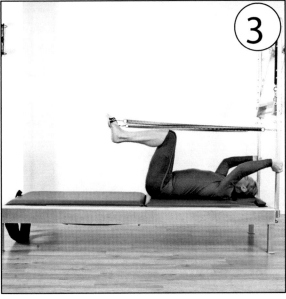

Setup:
Attach traditional leg springs with the Airplane Board at a height of 80 - 85 cm / 31.5 - 33.5 inches. The higher the spring attachment, the more the leg backsides have to work.

Supine position with the head pointing toward the spring attachments. The distance to the vertical bars of the Cadillac should be between half an arm-length and one arm-length. The further away, the harder the exercise. The hands hold the vertical bars slightly above the shoulders. Pelvis in a neutral position, spine in a natural position. Securely place the feet in the Airplane Board. The feet are slightly stretched. The legs are parallel and bent. The feet are slightly above the knees. The pelvis is neutral.

Purpose of the Exercise:
Mobilization of the hip.
Using the ischiocural musculature as movement initiators.
Strengthening of the hip and knee extensors.
Strengthening of the ankles and foot extensors.
Decoupling of the leg movement from the pelvis and trunk.

Execution: 5x - 10x
Stretch the legs gradually, resisting the spring force. The stability of the pelvis and the lower back is held. Bend the legs again and come back into the starting position.

Common Mistakes:
The pelvis tilts with the movement of the legs.
The knees are too far apart in the starting position.
The legs rotate inward while straightening.

Modifications or Variations:
For very tall people, the use of a loop with a longer loop or the use of an additional carabiner can lengthen the leg springs so that the force at the end of the movement is not too great.
Change of pace after the first five repetitions. First 5 slowly, then 5 faster.

Contraindications/Risks:
The exercise should be omitted in case of the following pre-existing conditions: acute herniated discs, listhesis of the lumbar spine, osteoporosis.

3. Dolphin & Dolphin Reverse (M)
1/2

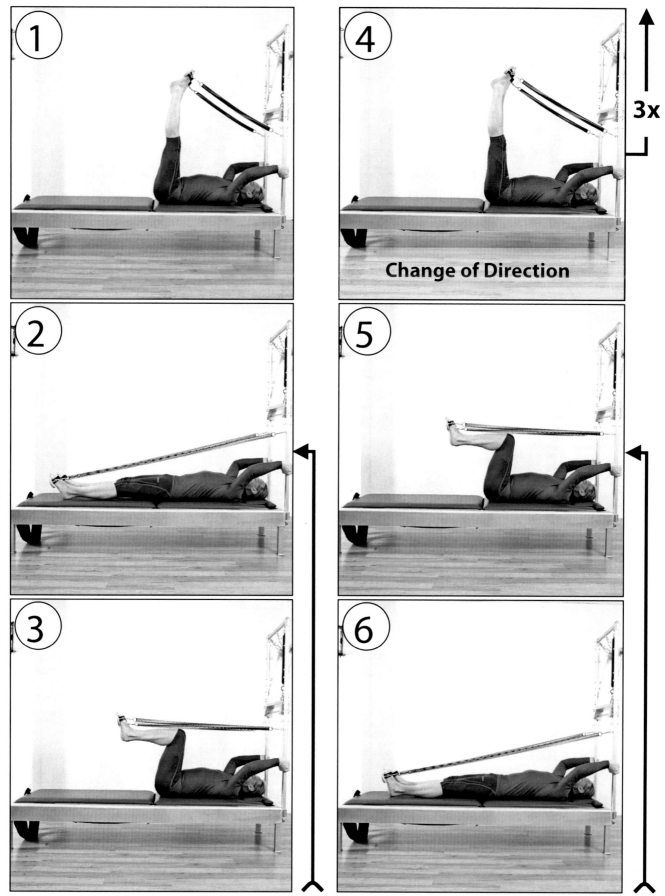

3x

Change of Direction

3. Dolphin & Dolphin Reverse (M)
2/2

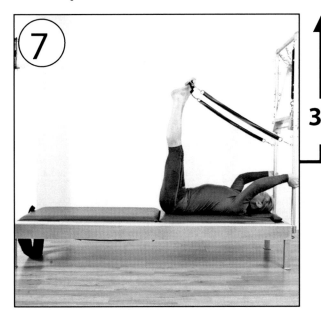

3x

Setup:

Attach traditional leg springs with the Airplane Board at a height of 80 - 85 cm / 31.5 - 33.5 inches. The higher the spring attachment, the more the leg backsides have to work.

Supine position with the head pointing toward the spring attachments. The distance to the vertical bars of the Cadillac should be between half an arm-length and one arm-length. The further away, the harder the exercise. The hands hold the vertical bars slightly above the shoulders. Pelvis in a neutral position, spine in a natural position. Securely place the feet in the Airplane Board. The feet are slightly stretched. The legs are parallel, closed and stretched up vertically with inner thigh tension. If the vertical position cannot be reached while maintaining a natural position of the spine (danger of a posterior pelvic tilt and strain on the lumbar spine), raise the legs only as far as the pelvis is stilly stable.

Purpose of the Exercise:

Mobilization of the hip.
Strengthening of the hip and knee extensors.
Decoupling the leg movement from the hip and torso.
Stretch of the leg backsides.

Execution: 5x - 10x per side

Image 2: Lower the stretched legs onto the Cadillac mat.
Image 3: Bring the legs into the tabletop position. Make sure to move the shins parallel to the Cadillac mat. Avoid excessively bending the knees. Imagine balancing a Box on the shins. Accordingly, the springs do not touch the legs.
Image 4: Stretch the legs upward. The knees remain in the same spot while straightening and are not
pulled   toward the chest.

Repeat 3x - 5x, then change the direction.

Image 5-6: From the table-top position, stretch the legs downward. Make sure to move the shins parallel to the Cadillac mat. Avoid excessively bending the knees.
Image 7: Move the stretched legs upward.

Repeat 3x - 5x.

Common Mistakes:

The stability of the pelvis is neglected.

Modifications or Variations: -

Contraindications/Risks: -

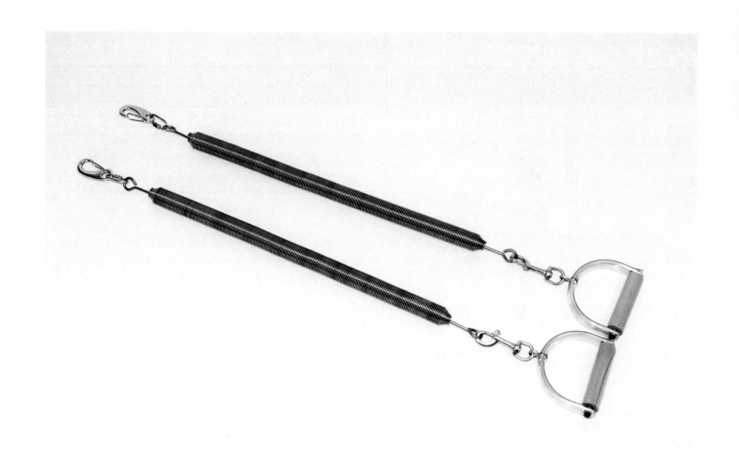

Arm Springs

Preliminary Remarks for the Arm Springs

The Arm Springs exercises are often performed at the Guillotine Tower. The advantage is that the Guillotine Tower has many metal hooks at different heights, so that the springs can be attached according to the height of the person. However, the Guillotine Tower can hardly still be found in studios nowadays, as it has to be mounted both to the floor and to the ceiling by an expert.

Balanced Body released a Guillotine Tower in 2016, which is attached to a supplied floor plate and may thus bring the Guillotine back to life.

In Pilates, there are often small series - as with the arm exercises. The typical beginners arm series while lying on the Cadillac consists of:

- Arm Up & Down

- Triceps

- Arm Circles

An advanced series while standing then consists of:

- Chest Expansion

- Squat

- Boxing

- Hug

- Shaving

- Bat / Butterfly

Beyond these exercises, however, there are many more exercises with the arm springs and, as always in Pilates, it is essential to find the exercises that are currently most helpful for the client.

Many different springs can be used for the arm exercises. Obviously, there is the standard arm spring from companies such as Gratz, Pilates Designs by Basil, etc., but many other springs work, too. Examples include the Baby/Arm Chair springs, yellow Balanced Body short and long springs, or Deborah Lessen Pilates Leg Springs which may also be used for arm work.

The appropriate exercise for the client at this moment, the correct spring, the correct height for the spring attachment, and the correct distance to the spring attachments determine to a large extent whether an exercise makes sense and can be performed successfully.

1. Up & Down (T)

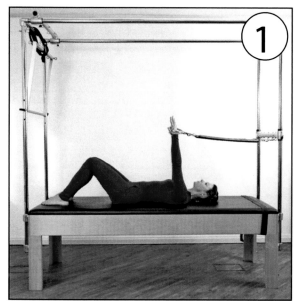

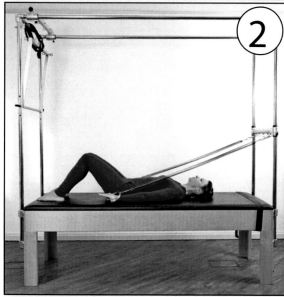

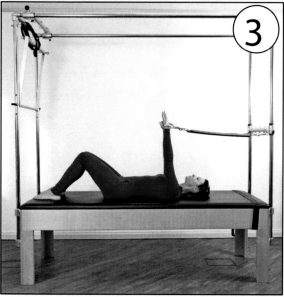

Setup:
Attach arm springs at a height of 55 cm / 21 inches. Supine position, with the head pointing toward the spring attachments and the legs standing on the mat. Select the distance and the springs so that the exercise can be performed completely without any evasive movements. The hands hold the handles, the fingers are as stretched as possible. The springs are not stretched yet but also do not hang loosely.

Purpose of the Exercise:
Strengthening of the latissimus dorsi, triceps and posterior part of the deltoideus.

Execution: 5x - 10x
Lower the stretched arms, keeping them close to the body. Hold for three seconds, then raise the arms again until the starting position is reached.

Common Mistakes:
During the downward movement, the shoulders round forward.
The arms rotate inward.
The arms are bent and the elbows drift outward.
The arms are moved outward instead of keeping them close to the body.

Modifications or Variations:
Change and adapt the height of the spring attachment.
Change and adapt the distance to the spring attachments.
Bring the legs into the tabletop position and pull the knees closer to the upper body, so that the thighs are no longer vertical but, instead, angled slightly further than 90 degrees. The aim is to activate the abdominal muscles.
In case the strength of the client has been overestimated, let the client push the arms down only as far as the movement can be performed without evasive movements, instead of changing the springs.

Contraindications/Risks:
In case of shoulder injuries, there is a risk of overstraining. In this case, use very light springs (Baby/Arm Chair Springs) and adapt the position so that the arm begins the movement already in or slightly higher than a 45 degree angle.

2.   Triceps (T)

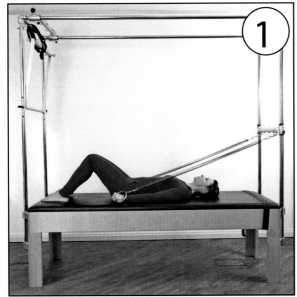

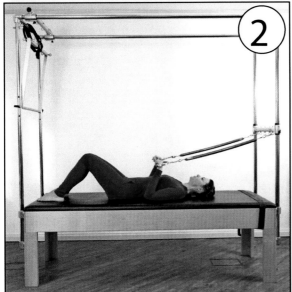

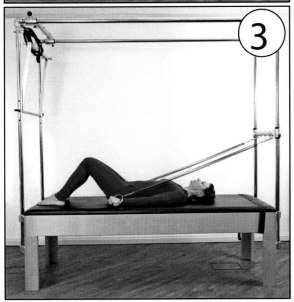

Setup:

Attach arm springs at a height of 55 cm / 21 inches.
Supine position, with the head pointing toward the spring attachments and the legs standing on the mat. Select the distance and the springs so that the exercise can be performed completely without any evasive movements. The hands hold the handles, the fingers are as stretched as possible. The position can be seen as a continuation of "Up and Down". After the last stretch of the arms, the bending begins. Hence, the arm already lies down completely and closely next to the body.

Purpose of the Exercise:

Strengthening of the triceps under the control of the arm adductors (M. triceps brachii (caput longum), M. latissimus dorsi, M. pectoralis major, M. teres major, M. teres minor, M. coracobrachialis).

Execution: 5x - 10x

Bend the lower arm, then stretch it again.

Common Mistakes:

The shoulders round forward.
The elbows evade the movement by moving to the sides.

Modifications or Variations:

Change and adapt the height of the spring attachment. Change and adapt the distance to the spring attachments.
Bring the legs into the tabletop position and pull the knees closer toward the upper body, so that the thighs are no longer vertical but, instead, angled slightly further than 90 degrees. The aim is to activate the abdominal muscles.
In case the arm cannot be stretched fully while the elbows touch the mat, the elbow can be raised slightly.

Contraindications/Risks:

In case of shoulder injuries, there is a risk of overstraining. In this case, use very light springs (Baby/Arm Chair Springs).

3. Supine Arm Circles (T)
1/3

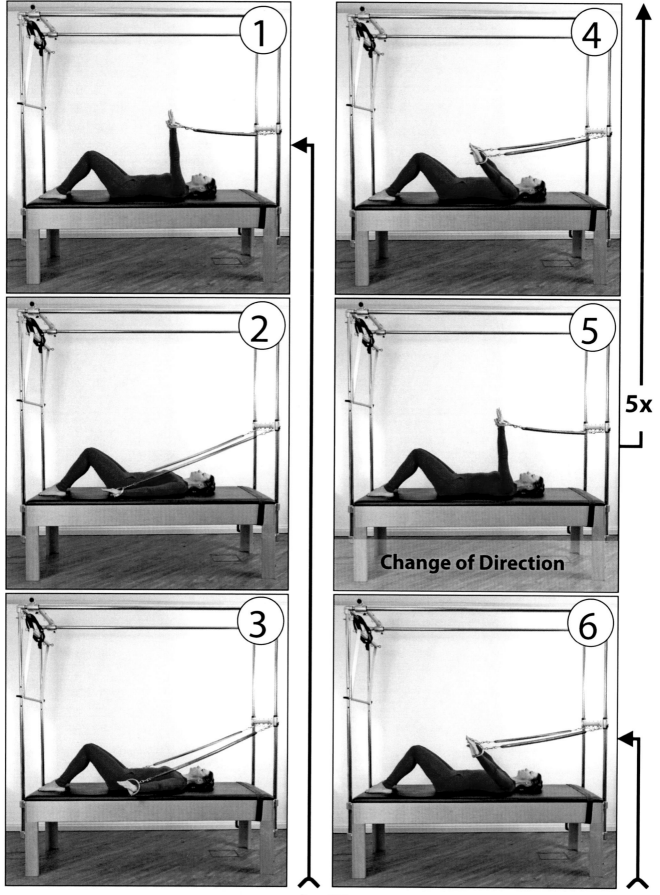

Change of Direction

5x

3. Supine Arm Circles (T)
2/3

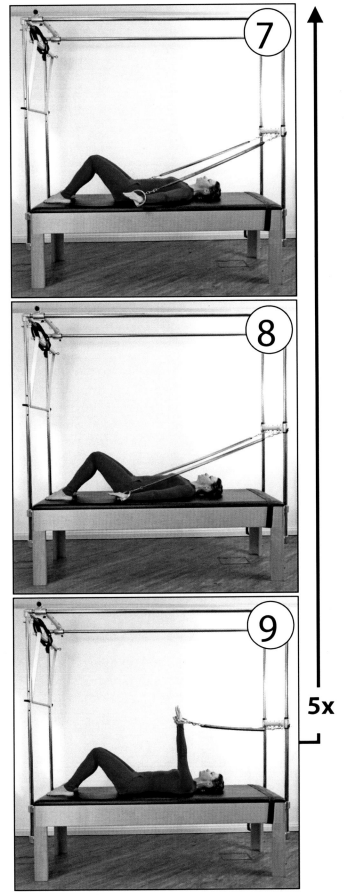

7

8

9

5x

3. Supine Arm Circles (T)
3/3

Setup:

Attach arm springs at a height of 55 cm / 21 inches. Supine position, with the head pointing toward the spring attachments and the legs standing on the mat. Select the distance and the springs so that the exercise can be performed completely without any evasive movements. The hands hold the handles, the fingers are as stretched as possible. The springs are not stretched yet but also do not hang loosely.

Purpose of the Exercise:

Stabilization of the shoulders.
Strengthening of the latissimus dorsi, triceps, posterior part of the deltoideus, pectoralis major, infraspinatus, and the biceps.

Execution: 5x - 10x per side

Lower the stretched arms, keeping them close to the body. From there, move the arms to the sides and then upward until the starting position is reached. The movement resembles a half-circle. After approx. 5 repetitions change the direction. The movement is performed evenly into all directions.

Common Mistakes:

During the downward movement, the shoulders round forward.
The arms rotate inward during the downward movement.
The arms are moved outward instead of keeping them close to the body during the downward movement.
The arms are bent and the elbows drift outward.
The arms are raised more quickly during the upward movement of the springs than they were moved downward against the spring force.
The control of the springs is given up at the end of the movement and, thus, "slam" at the highest point.

Modifications or Variations:

Change and adapt the height of the spring attachment.
Change and adapt the distance to the spring attachments.
Bring the legs into the tabletop position and pull the knees closer toward the upper body, so that the thighs are no longer vertical but, instead, angled slightly further than 90 degrees. The aim is to activate the abdominal muscles.
In case the strength of the client has been overestimated, let the client push the arms down only as far as the movement can be performed without evasive movements, instead of changing the springs.

Contraindications/Risks:

In case of shoulder injuries, there is a risk of overstraining. In this case, use very light springs (Baby/Arm Chair Springs) and adapt the position so that the arm begins the movement already in or slightly higher than a 45 degree angle.

4. Up & Down Advanced (T)

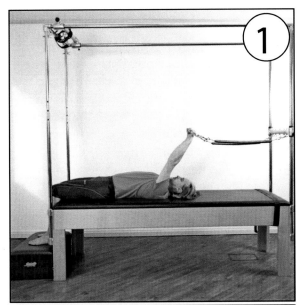

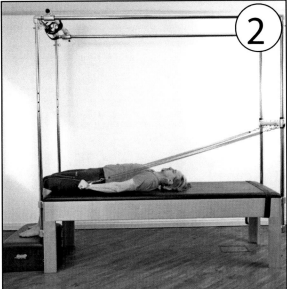

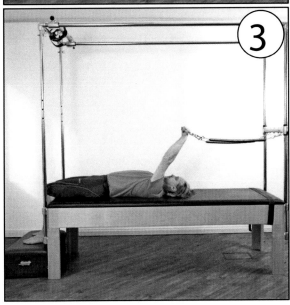

Setup:

Attach classic arm springs at a height of 55 cm / 21 inches. Supine position, with the head pointing toward the spring attachments. The hollows of the knees hang down from the opposite end of the Cadillac. The feet stand on a Reformer-Box. The hands hold the handles and form fists. The springs are not stretched yet but also do not hang loosely.

Purpose of the Exercise:

Strengthening of the latissimus dorsi, triceps and posterior part of the deltoideus.

Execution: 3x - 5x

Lower the stretched arms, keeping them close to the body. Hold for three seconds, then bring the arms back up until the starting position is reached.

Common Mistakes:

During the downward movement, the shoulders round forward. The arms rotate inward. The arms are bent and the elbows drift outward.

Modifications or Variations:

Choose the starting position closer to the spring attachments.
In case the strength of the client has been overestimated, let the client push the arms down only as far as the movement can be performed without evasive movements, instead of changing the springs.

Contraindications/Risks:

This is a very demanding exercise, which can lead to overstraining if not prepared sufficiently during the training.

5. Triceps Advanced (T)

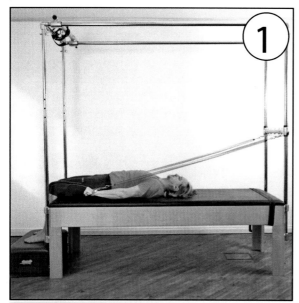

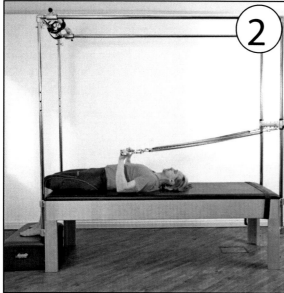

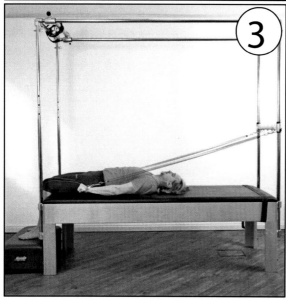

Setup:
Attach classic arm springs at a height of 55 cm / 21 inches.
Supine position, with the head pointing toward the spring attachments. The hollows of the knees hang down from the opposite end of the Cadillac. The feet stand on a Reformer-Box. The hands hold the handles and form fists. The setup position can be seen as a continuation of "Up and Down". After the last stretch of the arms, the bending begins. Hence, the arm already lies down completely and closely next to the body.

Purpose of the Exercise:
Strengthening of the triceps under the control of the arm adductors (M. triceps brachii (caput longum), M. latissimus dorsi, M. pectoralis major, M. teres major, M. teres minor, M. coracobrachialis).

Execution: 3x - 5x
Bend the lower arm and then stretch it again.

Common Mistakes:
The shoulders round forward.
The elbows evade the movement by moving to the sides.

Modifications or Variations:
In case the arm cannot be stretched fully while the elbows touch the mat, the elbow can be raised slightly. Choose the starting position closer to the spring attachments.

Contraindications/Risks:
This is a very demanding exercise, which can lead to overstraining if not prepared sufficiently during the training.

6. Supine Arm Circles Advanced (T)
1/3

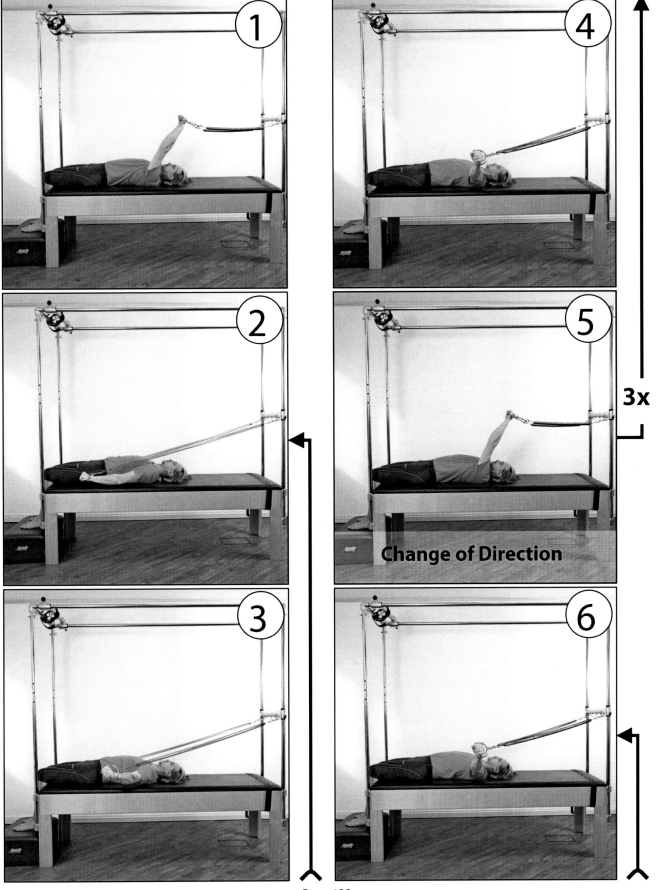

Change of Direction

3x

6. Supine Arm Circles Advanced (T)
2/3

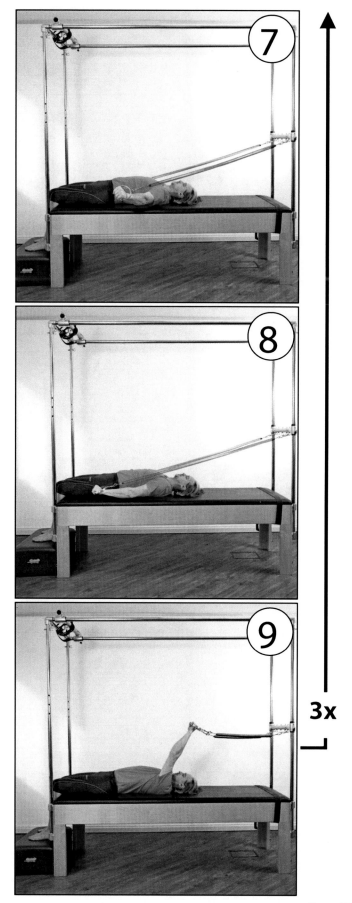

3x

6. Supine Arm Circles Advanced (T)
3/3

Setup:
Attach classic arm springs at a height of 55 cm / 21 inches.
Supine position, with the head pointing toward the spring attachments. The hollows of the knees hang down from the opposite end of the Cadillac. The feet stand on a Reformer-Box. The hands hold the handles and form fists. The springs are not stretched yet but also do not hang loosely.

Purpose of the Exercise:
Stabilization of the shoulders.
Strengthening of the latissimus dorsi, triceps posterior part of the deltoideus, deltoideus, pectoralis major, infraspinatus and the biceps.

Execution: 3x - 5x per side
Lower the stretched arms, keeping them close to the body. From there, bring them to the sides and finally back up until the starting position is reached. The movement resembles a half-circle. After 3 - 5 repetitions change the direction. The movement is performed evenly into all directions.

Common Mistakes:
During the downward movement, the shoulders round forward.
The arms rotate inward.
The arms are bent and the elbows drift outward.
The arms are moved outward instead of keeping them close to the body.
The arms are raised more quickly during the upward movement of the springs than they were moved downward against the spring force.
The control of the springs is given up at the end of the movement and, thus, "slam" at the highest point.

Modifications or Variations:
Choose the starting position closer to the spring attachments.
Change and adapt the height of the spring attachment.
In case the strength of the client has been overestimated, let the client push the arms down only as far as the movement can be performed without evasive movements, instead of changing the springs.

Contraindications/Risks:
This is a very demanding exercise, which can lead to overstraining if not prepared sufficiently during the training.

7. Chest Expansion Lunge (M)
1/2

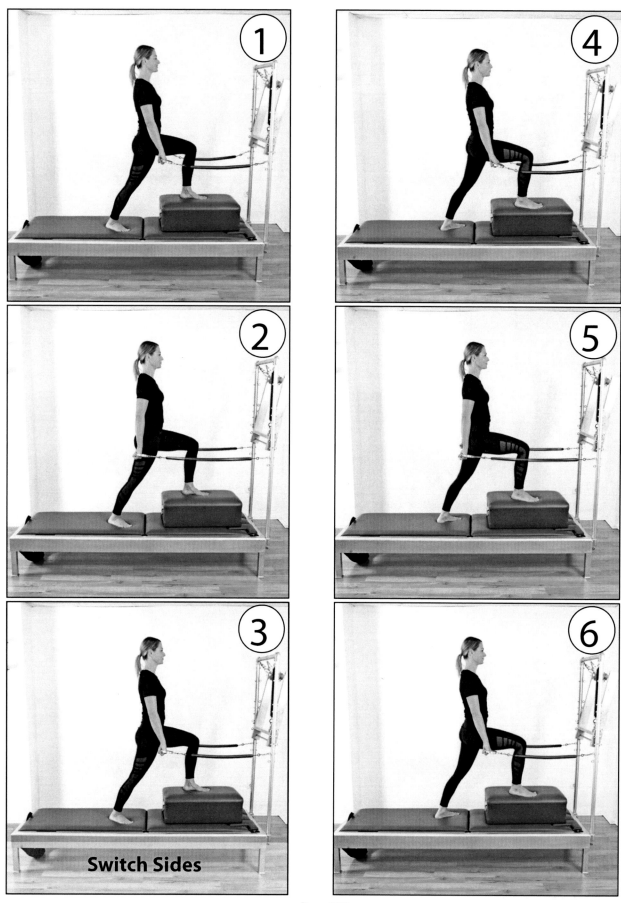

Switch Sides

7. Chest Expansion Lunge (M)
2/2

Setup:

Attach arm springs at a height of 55 cm / 21 inches.
Place a Reformer Box lengthwise on the Cadillac mat, close to the spring attachments.
Select the distance of the Box and of the body so that the exercise can be performed completely without any evasive movements. Standing in a small V on the Cadillac mat, looking toward the spring attachments. Place the left foot centrally on the Reformer-Box. The left knee is above the left ankle. The hands hold the handles, the fingers are as stretched as possible. The springs are not stretched yet but also do not hang loosely.

Purpose of the Exercise:

Strengthening of the latissimus dorsi, triceps and posterior part of the deltoideus.
Stretch.

Execution: 3x - 5x per leg position

Lower the stretched arms, keeping them close to the body. Hold for three seconds, then bring the arms back up and stretch them forward until the starting position is reached. The torso remains stable throughout the movement.

After 3-5 repetitions, switch sides and place the other leg on the Reformer-Box.

Common Mistakes:

The shoulders round forward during the back- and downward movement.
The arms rotate inward.
The arms are bent and the elbows drift outward.
The arms are moved outward instead of keeping them close to the body.

Modifications or Variations:

Attach the springs slightly above shoulder-height. Thereby the exercise becomes more demanding at the same distance from the spring attachments.
Change and adapt the distance to the spring attachments.

Contraindications/Risks: -

8. Chest Expansion with turn of head (T)
1/3

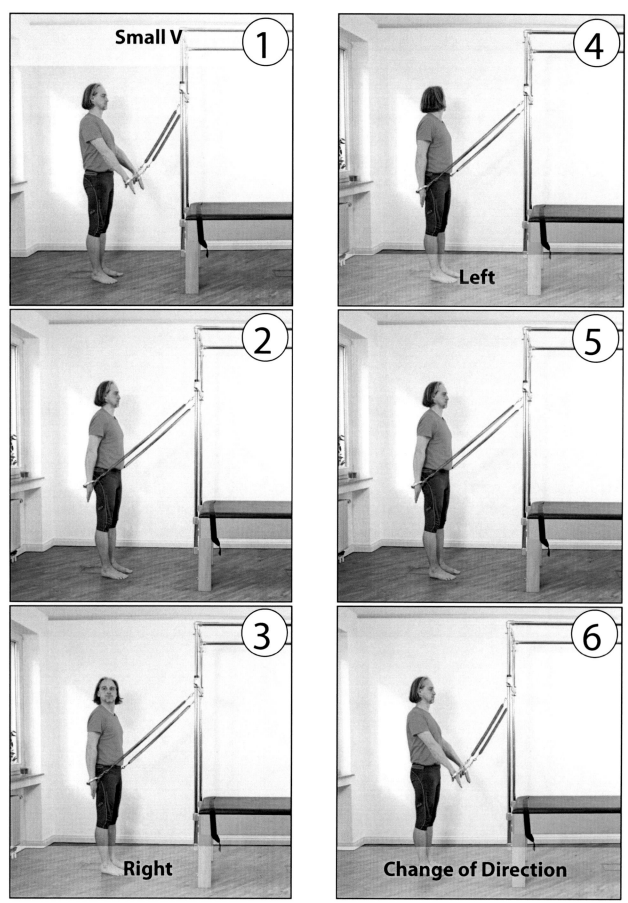

8. Chest Expansion with turn of head (T)
2/3

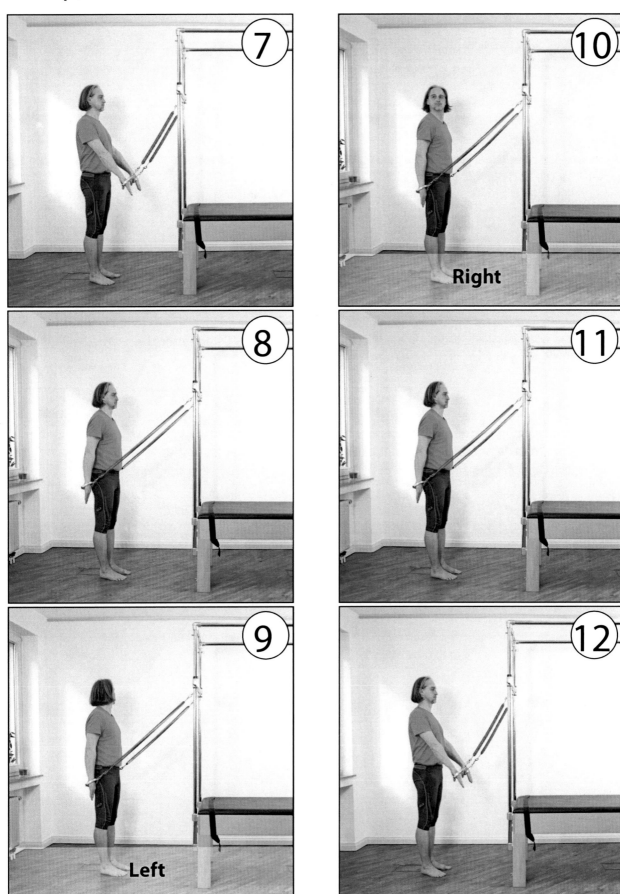

8. Chest Expansion with turn of head (T)
3/3

Setup:

Attach arm springs slightly above shoulder-height. Select the distance and the springs so that the exercise can be performed completely without any evasive movements. Standing in a small V outside the Cadillac, looking toward it. The hands hold the handles, the fingers are as stretched as possible. The springs are not stretched yet but also do not hang loosely.

Purpose of the Exercise:

Strengthening of the latissimus dorsi, triceps and posterior part of the deltoid.
Slight stretch of the anterior deltoid.
Stabilization of the torso through a strengthening of the long back extensors and the gluteal muscles.
Training the mobility of the cervical and upper thoracic spine.
Breathing exercise.

Execution: 4x - 6x

Inhaling, pull the arms backward, sideways past the body. Holding the breath, turn the head first to the right, then to the left and then to the center. While exhaling, bring the arms back until the spring is relaxed. Open the shoulders well throughout the movement and keep the torso upright. In order to optimize the rotation of the head, the shoulder depressors must work and the shoulder lifters must therefore be strained as little as possible. For the next repetition, start by turning the head to the left.

Common Mistakes:

The upper body sinks in and the shoulders are pulled forward, while the arms are rotated inward. In this case, turning the head is rather counterproductive.
The head is not rotated on one level, instead the chin is lowered during the rotation.
The arms are bent and the elbows drift outward.

Modifications or Variations:

Bring the arms behind the body. In this position, perform small pulses. Start with a pulse - and move your arms all the way back, then 1,2 pulses - and move the arms back, then 1,2,3 pulses - back. 1,2,3,4 - and so on with up to 10 pulses as the maximum. Then vice versa: 1,2,3,4,5,6,7,8,9 - and back. 1,2,3,4,5,6,7,8 - and back, and so on. Be careful, this modification is very intense.

Contraindications/Risks: -

9. Chest Expansion on Toes (T)
1/3

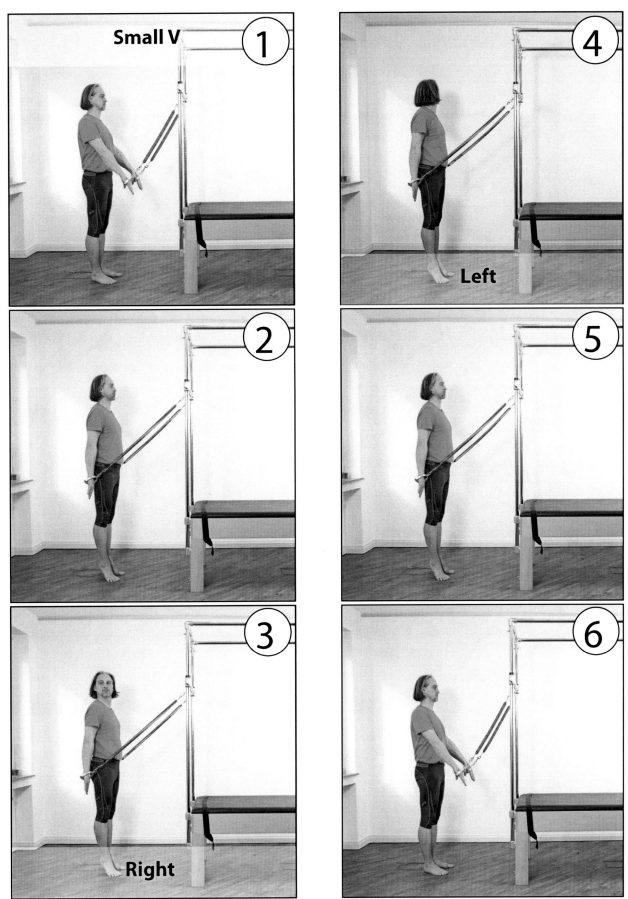

9. Chest Expansion on Toes (T)
2/3

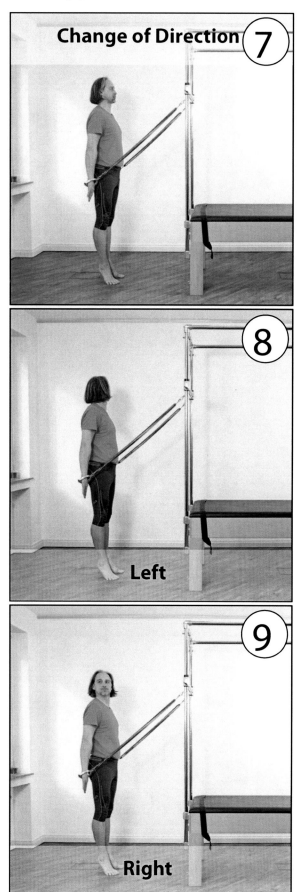

Change of Direction 7

8 Left

9 Right

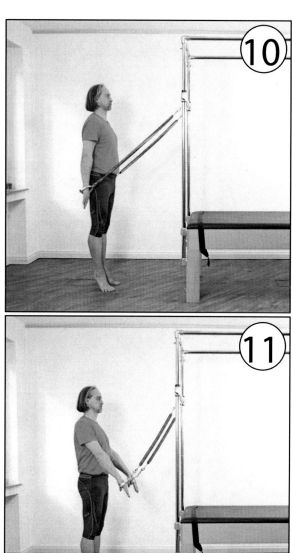

10

11

9. Chest Expansion on Toes (T)
3/3

Setup:

Attach arm springs slightly above shoulder-height.
Select the distance and the springs so that the exercise can be performed completely without any evasive movements. Standing in a small V outside the Cadillac, looking toward it. The hands hold the handles and the fingers are as stretched as possible. The springs are not stretched yet but also do not hang loosely.

Purpose of the Exercise:

Strengthening of the latissimus dorsi, triceps, posterior part of the deltoid and calf muscles.
Slight stretch of the anterior deltoid.
Stabilization of the torso by strengthening the long back extensors and the gluteal muscles.
Training the mobility of the cervical and upper thoracic spine.
Breathing and balancing exercise.

Execution: 4x - 6x

Inhaling, come up onto the tips of the toes without leaning forward any further. Then pull the arms backward, sideways past the body. Holding the breath, turn the head first to the right, then to the left and then to the center. While exhaling, bring the arms back until the spring is relaxed. Lower the heels again. Open the shoulders well throughout the movement and keep the torso upright. In order to optimize the rotation of the head, the shoulder depressors must work and the shoulder lifters must therefore be strained as little as possible. For the next repetition, start by turning the head to the left.

Common Mistakes:

The upper body sinks in and the shoulders are pulled forward, while the arms are rotated inward. In this case, turning the head is rather counterproductive.
The head is not rotated on one level, instead the chin is lowered during the rotation.
The arms are bent and the elbows drift outward.

Modifications or Variations:

Bring the arms behind the body. In this position, perform small pulses. Start with a pulse - and move your arms all the way back, then 1,2 pulses - and move the arms back, then 1,2,3 pulses - back. 1,2,3,4 - and so on with up to 10 pulses as the maximum. Then vice versa: 1,2,3,4,5,6,7,8,9 - and back. 1,2,3,4,5,6,7,8 - and back, and so on. Be careful, this modification is very intense.

Contraindications/Risks: -

10. Chest Expansion & Knee Bends (T)
1/2

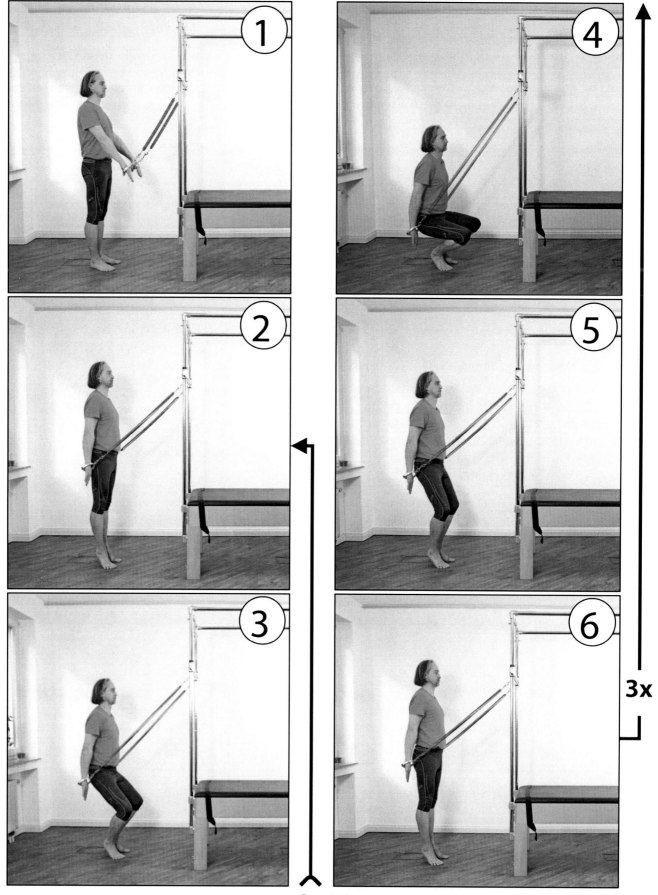

3x

10. Chest Expansion & Knee Bends (T)
2/2

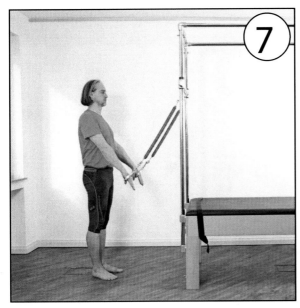

Setup:

Attach arm springs slightly above shoulder-height. Select the distance and the springs so that the exercise can be performed completely without any evasive movements. Standing in a small V outside the Cadillac, looking toward it. The hands hold the handles, the fingers are as stretched as possible. The springs are not stretched yet but also do not hang loosely.

Purpose of the Exercise:

Strengthening of the hip and knee flexors, knee extensors, ankles, latissimus dorsi, triceps and posterior deltoid.
Slight stretch of the anterior deltoid.
Stabilization of the torso by strengthening the long back extensors and the gluteal muscles.
Decoupling the leg movement from the hip and torso.
Breathing exercise.

Execution: 4x - 6x

Inhale, and come up onto the tips of the toes without leaning forward any further. Then pull the arms backward, sideways past the body. Hold the breath and bend the knees without changing the position of the arms and while keeping the back stretched. The knees move into the direction of and, if possible, beyond the second toe of each foot. Stretch the legs again. While exhaling, bring the arms back until the springs are relaxed. Keep the shoulders well-opened throughout the movement.
After the last repetition, lower the heels again.

Common Mistakes:

The upper body sinks in and the shoulders are pulled forward, while the arms are rotated inward.
The arms are bent and the elbows drift outward.
The knees are moved forward too straight, which unnecessarily strains the knee.

Modifications or Variations: -

Contraindications/Risks:

In case of knee endoprostheses, only indicate the knee flexion.

11. Chest Expansion & Squat (T)
1/4

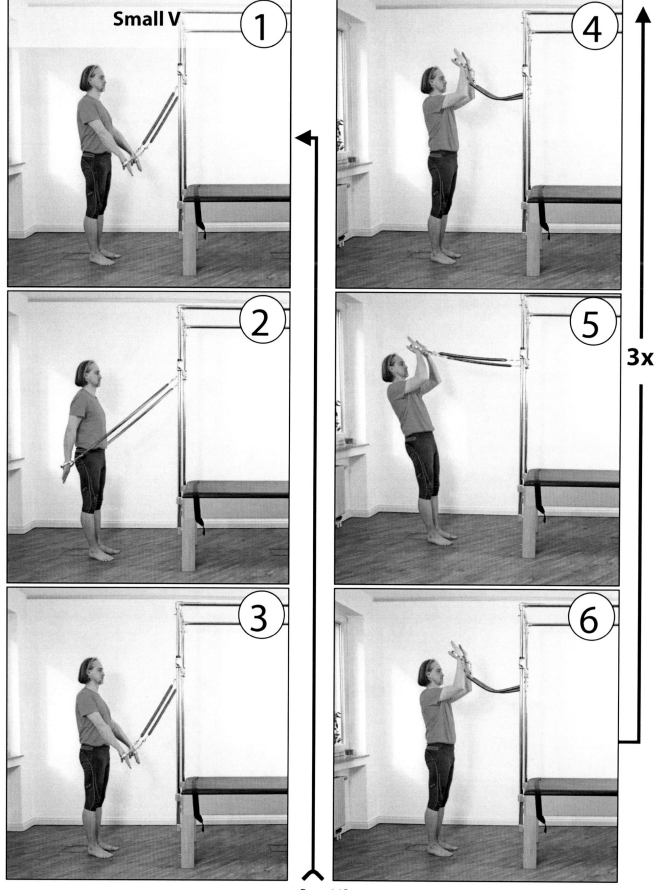

Small V

1

2

3

4

5

6

3x

11. Chest Expansion & Squat (T)
2/4

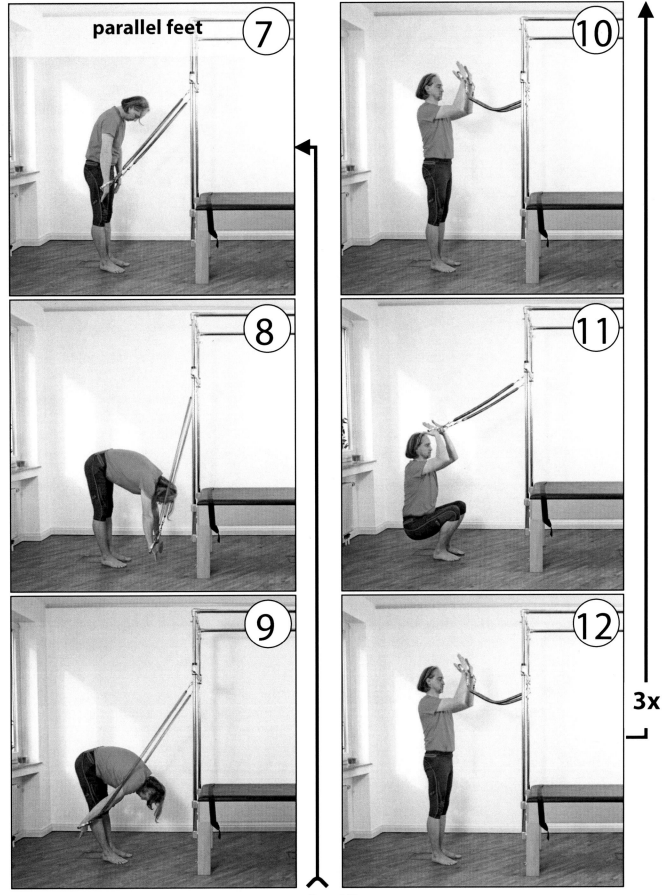

parallel feet

7

8

9

10

11

12

3x

11. Chest Expansion & Squat (T)
3/4

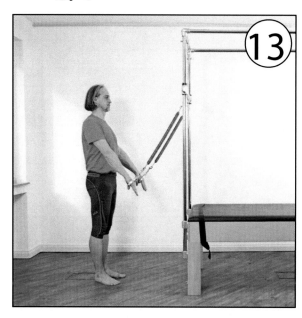

Setup:

Attach arm springs slightly above shoulder-height. Select the distance and the springs so that the exercise can be performed completely without any evasive movements. Standing in a small V outside the Cadillac, looking toward it. The hands hold the handles, the fingers are as stretched as possible. The springs are not stretched yet but also do not hang loosely.

Purpose of the Exercise:

Strengthening of the hip and knee extensors, ankles, latissimus dorsi, triceps and biceps brachii, and deltoideus. Slight stretch of the anterior deltoid in the arm extension. Stabilization of the torso by strengthening the long back extensors and the gluteal muscles.
Decoupling the leg movement from the hip and torso.

Execution: 3x - 5x per part

Part 1:

Image 2: Bring the arms backward, sideways past the body, until the springs are relaxed. Keep the shoulders well-opened throughout the movement.

Image 4: Rotate the arms until the hands face upward. Then bend the arms and raise them until the elbows are at shoulder height. Make sure that no complete 90 degree angle is reached so that the arms are still held by the back (latissimus dorsi).

Image 5-6: Lean the entire, stretched upper body backward. Form one long line from the ankle to the head. Do not change the arm position and maintain the arms' angle toward the upper body. Lean into the arm springs. Come back. Move the arms back into the starting position.

Repeat part 1 3x - 5x.

Part 2:

Image 7-9: Place the feet parallel to each other. Roll down and, with stretched arms, push the handles first downward and then toward the body and past the legs. Roll back up.

Image 10: Rotate the arms so that the hands face upward and then bend the arms, raising them until the elbows are at shoulder height. Make sure that no complete 90 degree angle is reached so that the arms are still held by the back (latissimus dorsi).

Image 11-12: Bend the knees without changing the position of the arms and while keeping the back stretched. The knees move forward straight across the center of the foot maximally up to the tips of the toes. Stretch the legs again. Move the arms back into the starting position.

Repeat part 2 3x - 5x.

11. Chest Expansion & Squat (T)
4/4

Common Mistakes:

The upper body sinks in and the shoulders are pulled forward, while the arms are rotated inward.
The arms are bent and the elbows drift outward.
The knees are moved beyond the tips of the toes, which unnecessarily strains the knee.
During the exercise, the arms are bent further than 90 degrees, bringing them closer to the head and causing the anterior chain to perform the holding work.

Modifications or Variations: -

Contraindications/Risks:

In case of knee endoprostheses, only indicate the knee flexion.

12. Chest Expansion Bottom Springs (T)
1/3

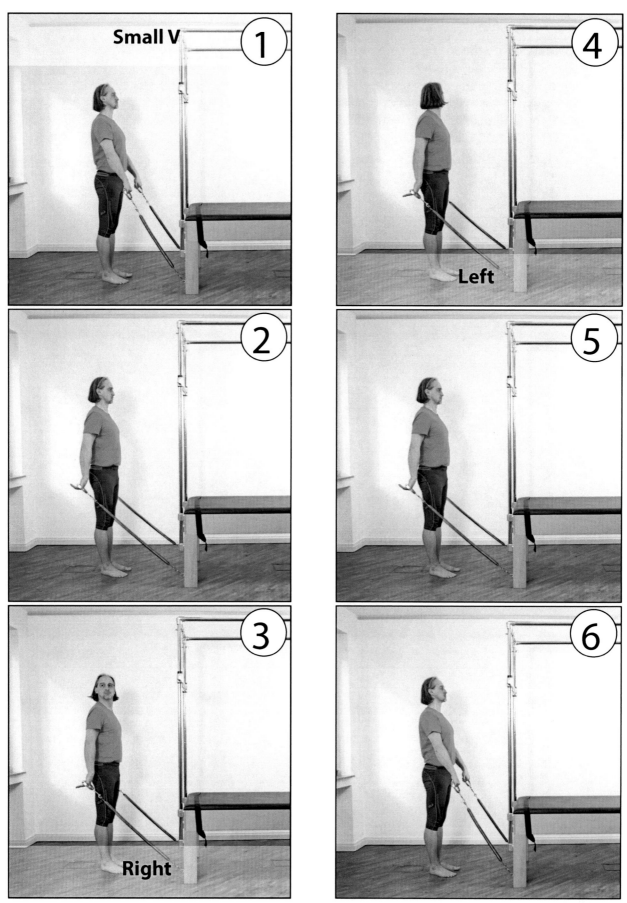

12. Chest Expansion Bottom Springs (T)
2/3

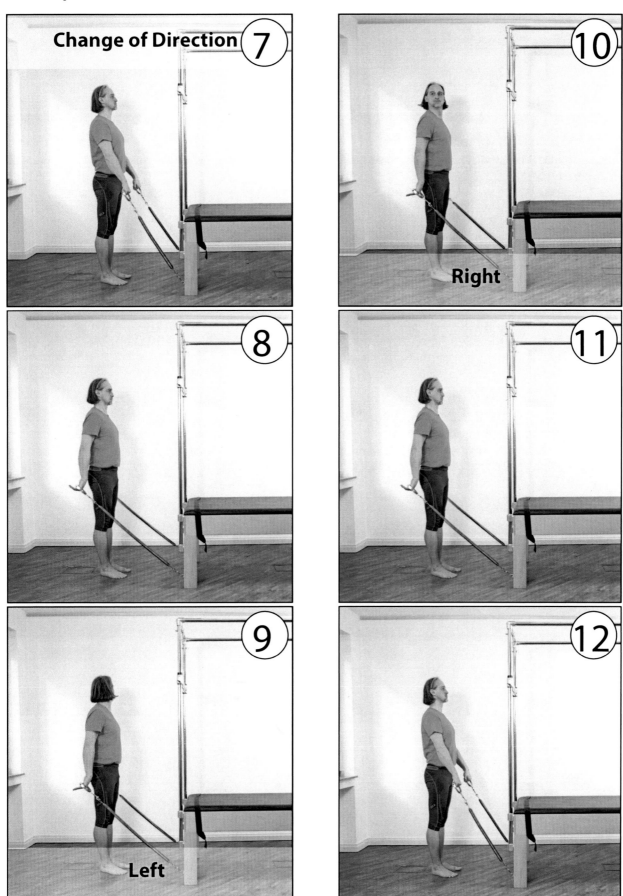

12. Chest Expansion Bottom Springs (T)
3/3

Setup:

Attach arm springs at the lowest point of the Cadillac. Select the distance and the springs so that the exercise can be performed completely without any evasive movements. Standing in a small V outside the Cadillac, looking toward it. The hands hold the handles, the fingers are as stretched as possible. The springs are not stretched yet but also do not hang loosely.

Purpose of the Exercise:

Strengthening of the latissimus dorsi, triceps and posterior part of the deltoid.
Slight stretch of the anterior deltoid.
Stabilization of the torso by strengthening the long back extensors and the gluteal muscles.
Training the mobility of the cervical and upper thoracic spine.
Breathing exercise.

Execution: 4x - 6x

Exhale and pull the arms backward, sideways past the body. Holding the breath, turn the head first to the right, then to the left and then to the center. While exhaling, bring the arms back until the spring is relaxed. Open the shoulders well throughout the movement and keep the torso upright. In order to optimize the rotation of the head, the shoulder depressors must work and the shoulder lifters must therefore be strained as little as possible. For the next repetition, start by turning the head to the left.

Common Mistakes:

The upper body sinks in and the shoulders are pulled forward, while the arms are rotated inward. In this case, turning the head is rather counterproductive.
The head is not rotated on one level, instead the chin is lowered during the rotation.
The arms are bent and the elbows drift outward.

Modifications or Variations:

Bring the arms behind the body. In this position, perform small pulses. Start with a pulse - and move your arms all the way back, then 1,2 pulses - and move the arms back, then 1,2,3 pulses - back. 1,2,3,4 - and so on with up to 10 pulses as the maximum. Then vice versa: 1,2,3,4,5,6,7,8,9 - and back. 1,2,3,4,5,6,7,8 - and back, and so on. Be careful, this modification is very intense.

Contraindications/Risks: -

13. Standing Hug (T)
1/2

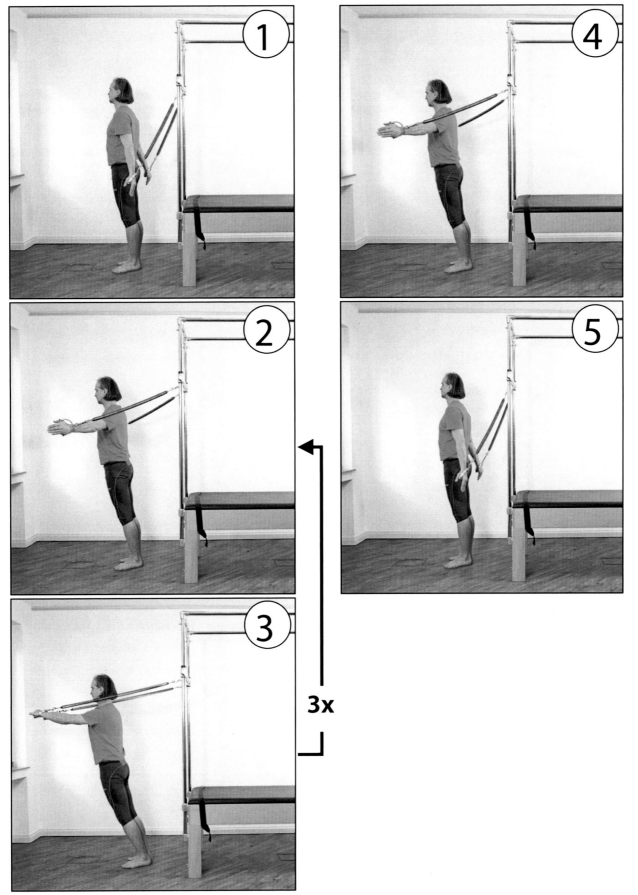

3x

13. Standing Hug (T)
2/2

Setup:

Attach arm springs slightly above shoulder-height. Select the distance and the springs so that the exercise can be performed completely without any evasive movements. Standing in a small V outside the Cadillac, looking away from it. The hands hold the handles, the fingers are stretched. The springs are not stretched yet but also do not hang loosely. Bring the arms up until slightly below shoulder-height, stretched to the sides.

Purpose of the Exercise:

Strengthening of the pectoralis major.
Stabilization of the shoulders and entire torso musculature. Full body tension.

Execution: 3x - 5x

Move the arms toward each other in front of the body. The elbows are bent very slightly. The hands shortly touch each other with the fingertips before opening the arms to the sides again.

After 3-5 repetitions lower the arms to the body sides again.

Common Mistakes:

The distance was chosen incorrectly and the body loses its stability during the exercise.
Leaning forward in the hip with the forward movement of the arms. As a whole, the body forms a large "C". The stability of the scapulae is given up and they constantly move. There is often an excessive protraction of the scapulae during the forward movement of the arms.
A mistake is made while coming back, as the two springs are brought into the neutral position one after the other (click/clack instead of a joint clack).
The shoulders round as the arms are moved forward, the chest sinks in and the stability of the scapulae is lost.
The tightening of the ribs through the external abdominal muscles is lost as the arms are moved back to the sides.

Modifications or Variations:

Using a higher spring attachment.
The hands form fists for a stronger focus on the strength-aspect of the exercise.
A variation to target the different parts of the pectoralis: The hands point downward slightly. During the movement of the arms toward each other, the thumbs meet first. During the second meeting, the index fingers touch, and so on, until the little fingers touch. On the way from the thumb to the little finger, the hands gradually rotate with each repetition until they point slightly upward.

Contraindications/Risks: -

14. Boxing (T)
1/3

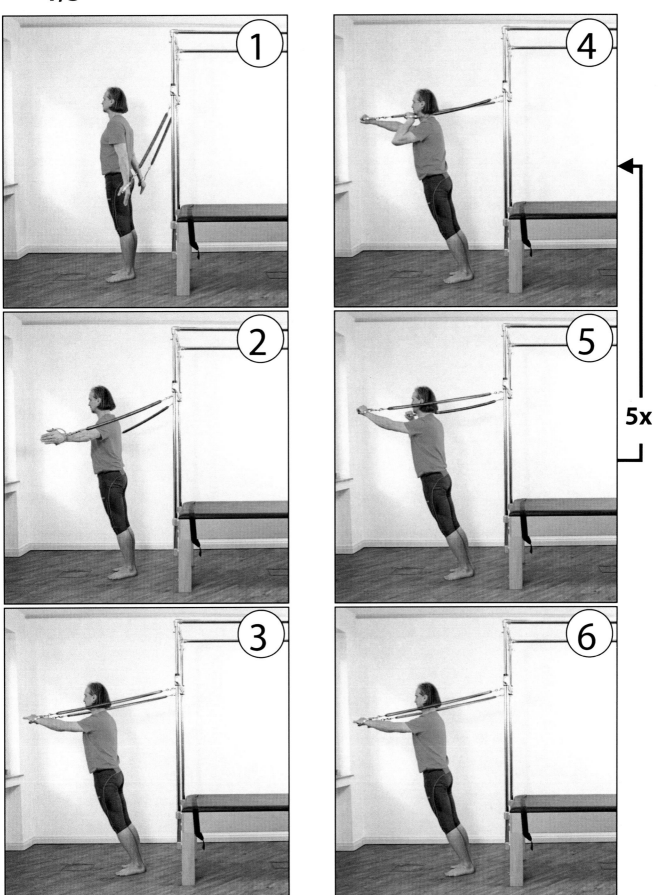

14. Boxing (T)
2/3

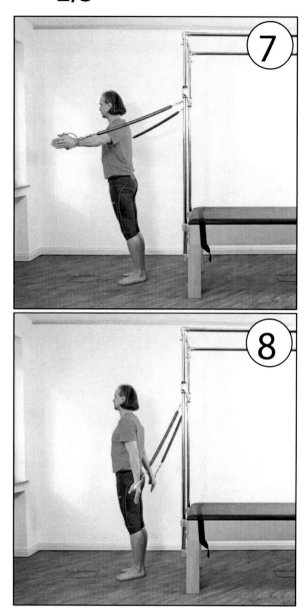

14. Boxing (T)
3/3

Setup:

Attach arm springs slightly above shoulder-height. Select the distance and the springs so that the exercise can be performed completely without any evasive movements. Standing in a small V outside the Cadillac, looking away from it. The hands hold the handles, the fingers are stretched. The springs are not stretched yet but also do not hang loosely. Bring the arms up until slightly below shoulder-height, stretched to the sides. Then bring them together in front of the body as in the Hug and come slightly above the shoulders. The hands form fists.

Purpose of the Exercise:

Strengthening of the pectoralis major pars clavicularis and sternalis, anterior part of the deltoid and the triceps.
Stabilization of the abdominal muscles. Full body tension.

Execution: 5x - 10x per side

Move one arm back to the face. The fist is approx. at chin-height. The elbows constantly remain at shoulder-height. This fist is moved forward in a straight line while the other is brought backward.

Box 5-10x per side, then bring both hands forward. Open the fists and move the arms back as in the Hug. Then let both arms sink down on the sides.

Common Mistakes:

The distance was chosen incorrectly and the body loses its stability during the exercise.
Leaning forward in the hip with the forward movement of the arms. As a whole, the body forms a large "C". The upper body rotates along with the Boxing movement.
The stability of the scapulae is given up and they constantly move. There is often an excessive protraction of the scapulae while straightening the arms.
The elbow sinks during the backward movement.
The arm that is moved forward is not stretched fully.
The arm that is moved forward is locked into place in the joint in front of the body, instead of performing a continuous forward movement all the way to the turning point.
The torso does not remain stable and rotates instead. The upper body follow the forward movement of the arms.
A mistake is made while coming back, as the two springs are brought into the neutral position one after the other (click/clack instead of a joint clack).

Modifications or Variations:

Using a higher spring attachment.
Box higher up, like having a taller opponent.

Contraindications/Risks: -

15. Boxing in 8 counts (T)
1/4

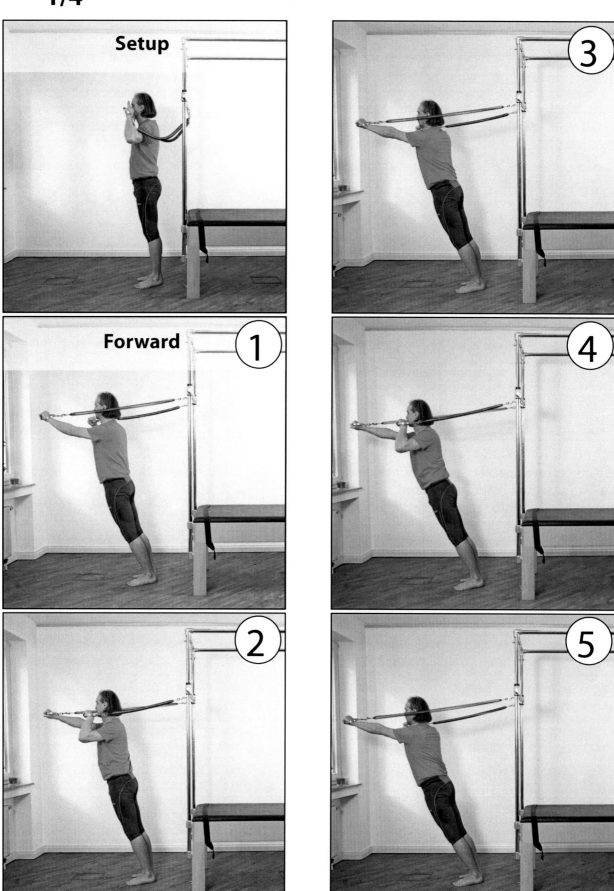

Setup

Forward ①

②

③

④

⑤

15. Boxing in 8 counts (T)
2/4

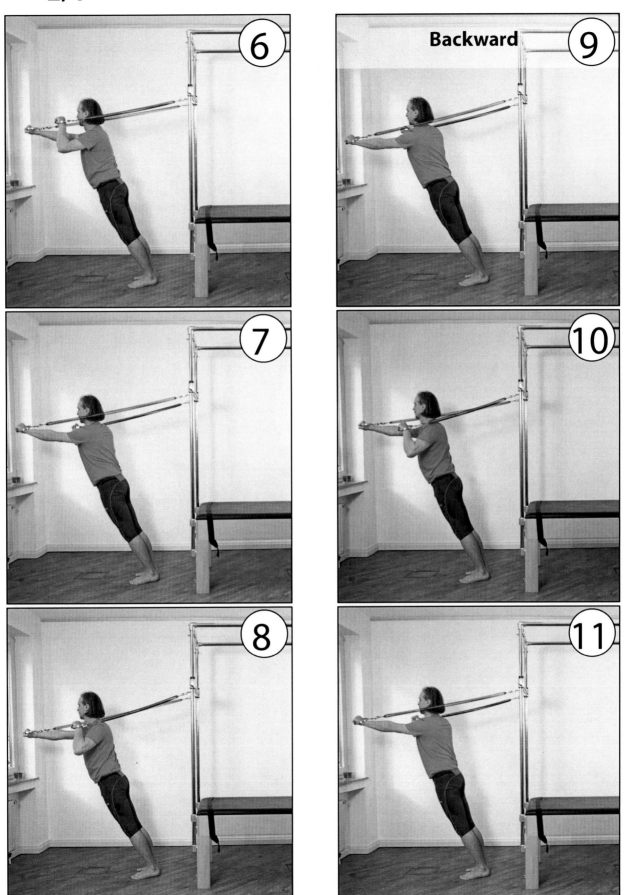

15. Boxing in 8 counts (T)
3/4

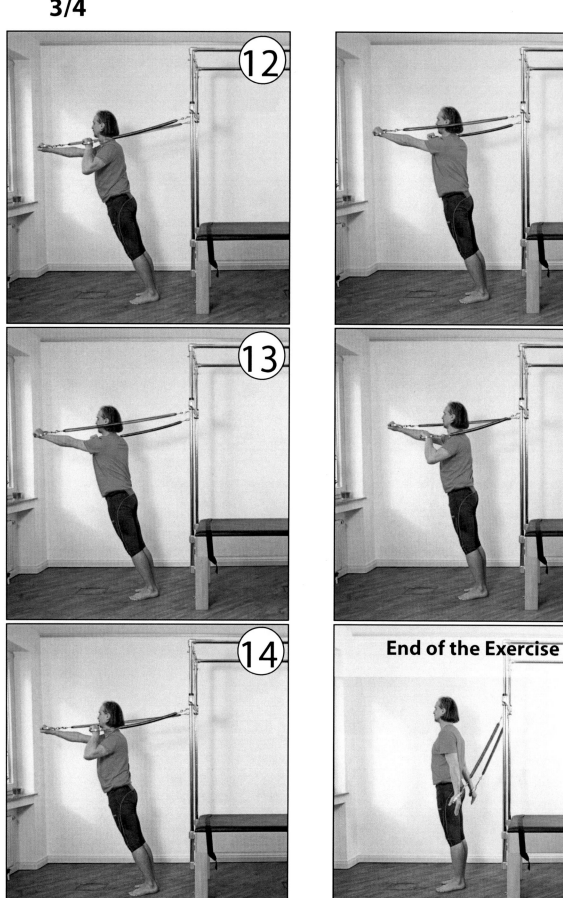

15. Boxing in 8 counts (T)
4/4

Setup:

Attach classic arm springs slightly above shoulder-height. Select the distance so that the exercise can be performed completely without any evasive movements. Standing in a small V outside the Cadillac, looking away from it. The hands hold the handles, the fingers are stretched. The springs are not stretched yet but also do not hang loosely. Bring the arms up until slightly below shoulder-height, stretched to the sides. Then bring them together in front of the body as in the Hug and come slightly above the shoulders. The hands form fists.

Purpose of the Exercise:

Strengthening of the pectoralis major pars clavicularis and sternalis, anterior part of the deltoid, triceps brachii and serratus anterior.
Stabilization of the abdominal muscles. Fully body tension.

Execution: 5x - 10x per side

Move one arm back to the face. The fist is approx. at chin-height. The elbows constantly remain at shoulder-height. This fist is moved forward in a straight line while the other is brought backward. During each punch lean forward more and more without rotating along.
After 8 punches, come back the same way.

Repeat this sequence 1-5x. Then bring both hands to the front. Open the fists and move the arms back as in the Hug. Then let both arms sink down on the sides.

Common Mistakes:

The distance was chosen incorrectly and the body loses its stability during the exercise.
Leaning forward in the hip with the forward movement of the arms. As a whole, the body forms a large "C".
The upper body rotates along with the Boxing movement.
The stability of the scapulae is given up and they constantly move. There is often an excessive protraction of the scapulae while straightening the arms.
The elbow sinks during the backward movement.
The arm that is moved forward is not stretched fully.
The arm that is moved forward is locked into place in the joint in front of the body, instead of performing a continuous forward movement all the way to the turning point.
The torso does not remain stable and rotates instead. The upper body follow the forward movement of the arms.
A mistake is made while coming back, as the two springs are brought into the neutral position one after the other (click/clack instead of a joint clack).

Modifications or Variations: -

Contraindications/Risks:

Caution: Danger of falling.

16. Fencing (T)
1/2

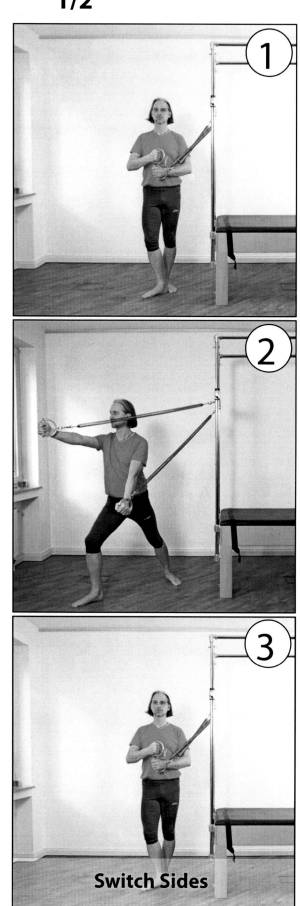

Switch Sides

16. Fencing (T)
2/2

Setup:

Attach arm springs slightly above shoulder-height. Select the distance and the springs so that the exercise can be performed completely without any evasive movements. Standing sideways in a small V, next to the Cadillac. Slide the outer foot (farther away from the Cadillac) forward along the inner foot until the heel of the outer foot touches the big toe of the inner foot. The outer foot forms a right angle with the inner foot. The hands hold the handles and form fists. The outer arm holds the anterior spring. The inner arm holds the rear spring. Both hands are below the chest. The outer fist is above the inner fist.

Purpose of the Exercise:

Strengthening of the deltoid, pectoralis major, triceps brachii, and serratus anterior.
Stabilization of the entire abdominal and back musculature. Transverse tension of the whole body.

Execution: 3x - 6x per side

Fast, powerful lunge at a 45 degree angle. Simultaneously bring the upper arm (right arm in the image) forward at a 45 degree angle. Relative to the upper body, this arm is stretched outward only slightly more than 90 degrees. Looking in the direction of the upper punching hand. The inner arm (left arm in the image) moves downward and forward at the same time as if it was defending a punch with a shield. Come back with a powerful, springy step.

Perform 3x - 6x per side, then switch sides.

Common Mistakes:

Instead of 45 degrees, the punch of the upper arm is performed in a straight line away from the Cadillac. The spring then nearly touches the face.

Modifications or Variations:

Alternatively, the lower arm is not stretched but bent (soft elbow), as if it was defending a punch with a shield.

Contraindications/Risks: -

17. Rowing Standing (T)
1/3

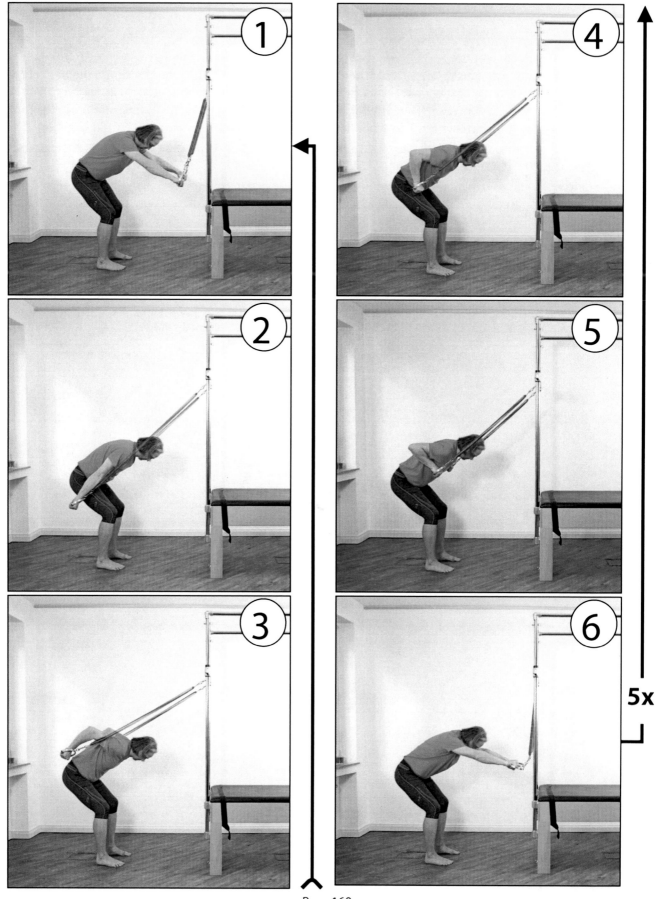

5x

17. Rowing Standing (T)
2/3

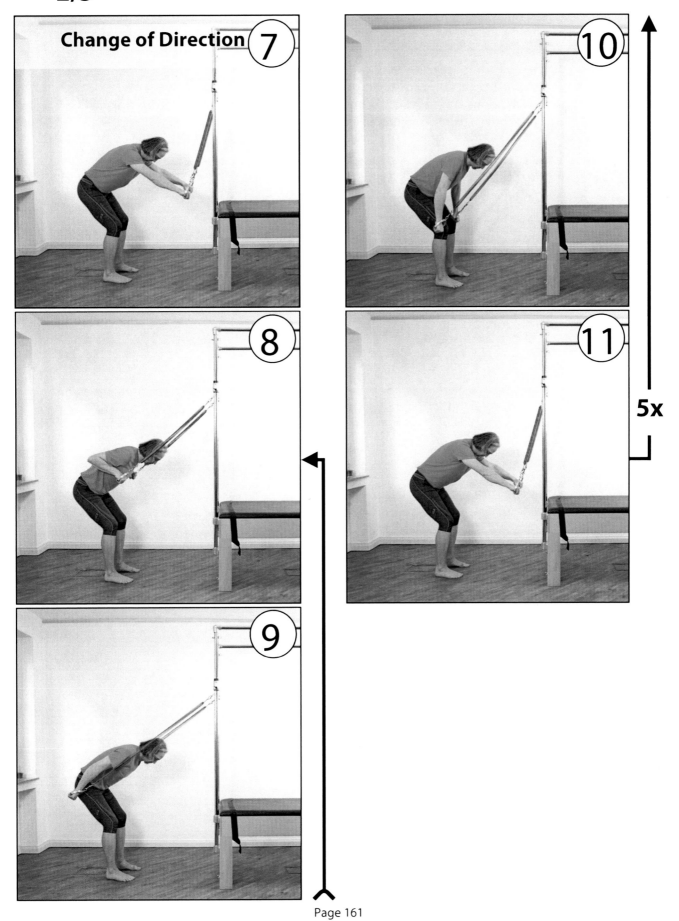

Change of Direction

7

8

9

10

11

5x

17. Rowing Standing (T)
3/3

Setup:

Attach arm springs slightly above shoulder-height. Select the distance and the springs so that the exercise can be performed completely without any evasive movements.

Standing with the feet parallel and hip-wide apart outside the Cadillac, looking toward it. The hands hold the handles and form fists. The arms are stretched. Bent legs. The upper body forms a C-curve. The head follows the flexion of the upper body, looking at the ground right in front of the feet.

Purpose of the Exercise:

Strengthening of the latissimus dorsi, triceps and posterior part of the deltoid.
Slight stretch of the anterior deltoid.
Stabilization of the entire abdominal musculature, pelvic floor and leg muscles.

Execution: 5x - 10x per direction

Bring both arms downward in a straight line and then parallel to the upper body. Then bend the elbows parallel to each other and move them upward. Move the hands along the torso to the armpits and from there stretch the arms back out to the front. The forearms and hands rotate outward where necessary in the exercise to minimize the contact with the springs.

After 5-10 repetitions change the direction.

Bend both elbows parallel to each other and pull them backward, past the body. Then stretch the arms out down- and backward completely. Move the stretched arms to the front in a parallel motion. The forearms and hands rotate outward where necessary in the exercise to minimize the contact with the springs.

Repeat 5-10x.

Common Mistakes:

Bending the upper body too far forward, until it is almost parallel to the floor.
The elbows move into opposite directions during the backward pulling movement.
The rowing movement is too small, the arms are never fully stretched.

Modifications or Variations: -

Contraindications/Risks: -

18. Rowing Standing Reverse (T)
1/3

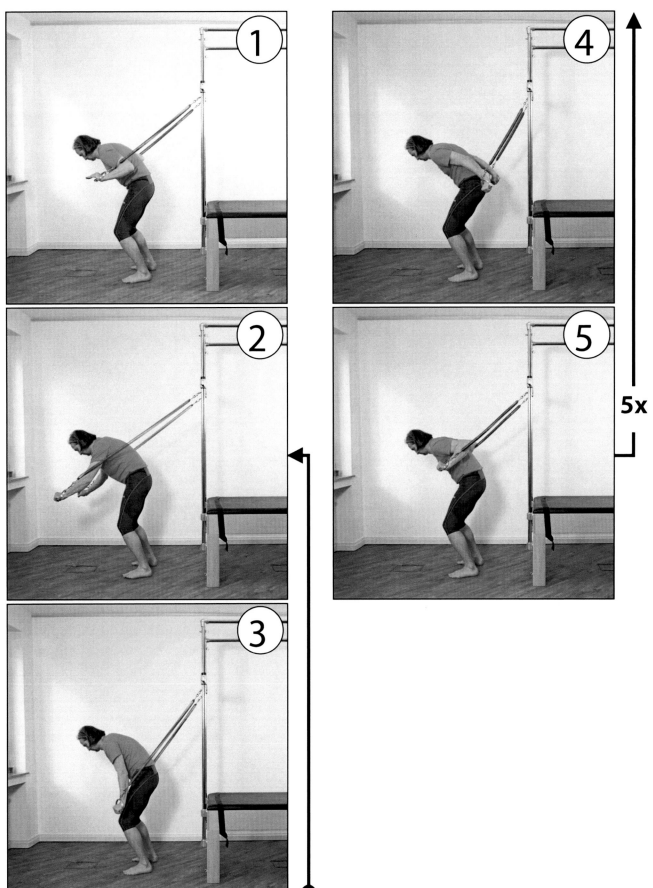

5x

18. Rowing Standing Reverse (T)
2/3

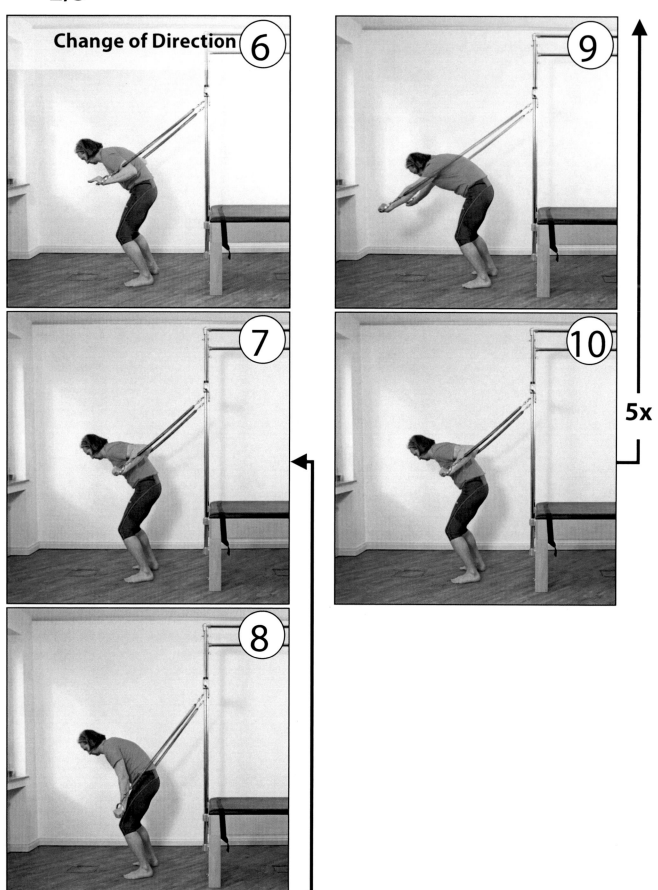

Change of Direction

5x

18. Rowing Standing Reverse (T)
3/3

Setup:
Attach arm springs slightly above shoulder-height. Select the distance and the springs so that the exercise can be performed completely without any evasive movements. Standing with the feet parallel and hip-wide apart outside the Cadillac, looking away from it. The hands hold the handles and form fists. The arms are bent. The springs come from above. Bent legs. The upper body forms a C-curve. The head follows the flexion of the upper body, looking at the ground right in front of the feet.

Purpose of the Exercise:
Strengthening of the pectoralis major pars clavicularis and sternalis, anterior part of the deltoid, triceps brachii and serratus anterior.
Stabilization of the entire abdominal musculature, the pelvic floor and the leg muscles.

Execution: 5x - 10x per direction
Bring both arms downward in a straight line and then parallel to the upper body. Then bend the elbows parallel to each other and move them upward. Move the hands along the torso to the armpits and from there stretch the arms back to the front. The forearms and hands rotate outward where necessary in the exercise to minimize the contact with the springs.

After 5-10 repetitions change the direction.

Bend both elbows in a parallel motion and pull them backward, past the body. Then stretch the arms out down- and backward completely. Move the stretched arms to the front parallel. The forearms and hands rotate outward where necessary in the exercise to minimize the contact with the springs.

Repeat 5-10x.

Common Mistakes:
Bending the upper body too far forward, until it is almost parallel to the floor.
The elbows move into opposite directions during the backward pulling movement.
The rowing movement is too small.

Modifications or Variations: -
Slightly rotate the forearms outward.

Contraindications/Risks: -

19. Squat with one leg (T)
1/3

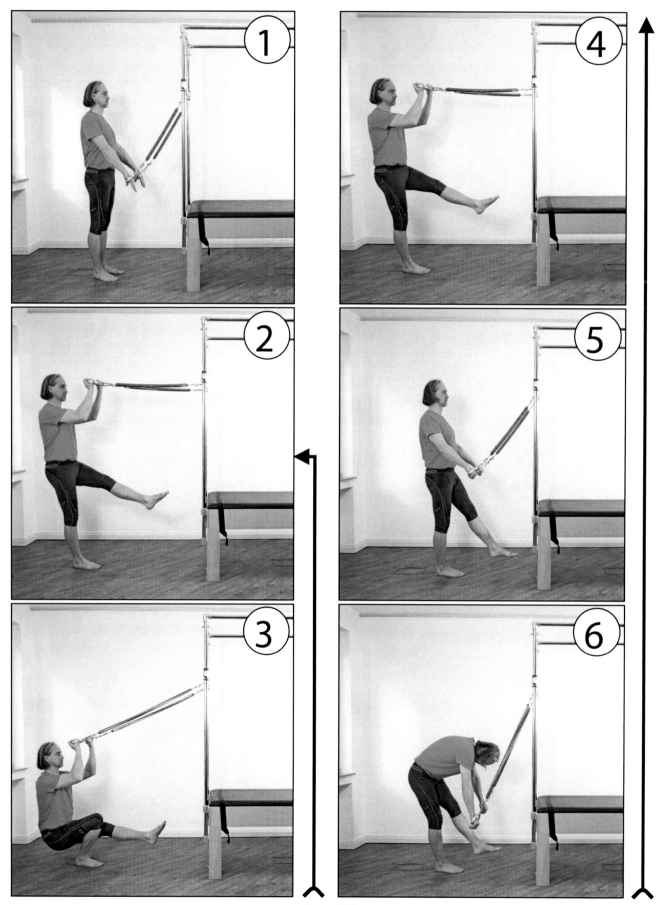

19. Squat with one leg (T)
2/3

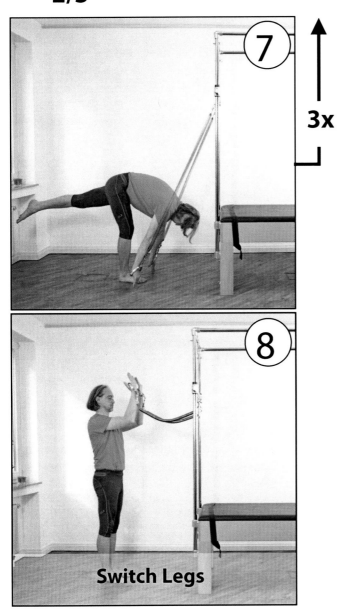

3x

Switch Legs

19. Squat with one leg (T)
3/3

Setup:

Attach arm springs slightly above shoulder-height. Select the distance and the springs so that the exercise can be performed completely without any evasive movements. Standing with parallel feet outside the Cadillac, looking toward it. The feet are one foot-width apart. The hands hold the handles and face backward, the fingers are as stretched as possible. The springs are not stretched yet but also do not hang loosely.

Purpose of the Exercise:

Strengthening of the latissimus dorsi, triceps and posterior part of the deltoid.
Slight stretch of the anterior deltoid.
Stabilization of the torso by strengthening the long back extensors and the gluteal muscles.
Strengthening of the hip flexors, knee extensors and ankles.
Decoupling the leg movement from the hip and torso.

Execution: 3x - 5x per side

Rotate the arms so that the hands point upward and then flex the arms so that the elbows are at shoulder level. Make sure that no complete 90 degree angle is reached so that the arms are held by the back (latissimus dorsi). Raise one leg.
Bend the knee of the standing leg without changing the position of the arms and while keeping the back stretched. The knee of the standing leg moves straight forward to the center of the foot, maximally up to the tips of the toes. The height of the bending is very individual. The heel of the standing leg remains in touch with the ground.
Then stretch the leg again.
Now bring the arms back into the starting position in front of the body.
Roll down and push the handles down with stretched arms first and then into the direction of the standing leg. The leg, which was stretched forward before, is now brought backward. During the movement, look at the foot.
Roll back up and put the legs down next to each other. Switch legs.

Common Mistakes:

The upper body sinks in and the shoulders are pulled forward, while the arms are rotated inward.
The arms are bent and the elbows drift outward.
The knee of the standing leg is moved beyond the tips of the toes, which unnecessarily strains it.
During the exercise, the arms are bent further than 90 degrees, bringing them closer to the head and causing the anterior chain to perform the holding work.

Modifications or Variations: -

Contraindications/Risks: -

20. Lunges (T)
1/2

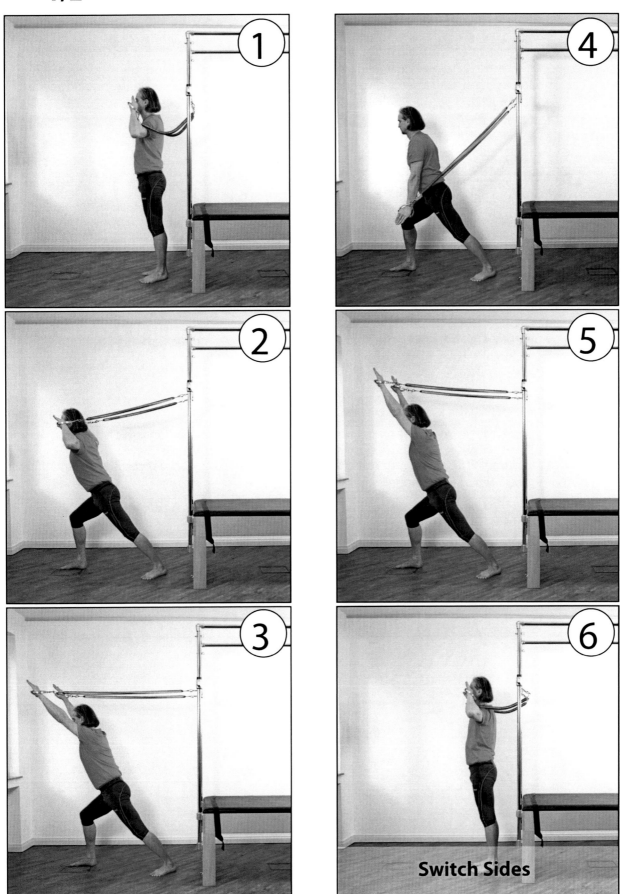

20. Lunges (T)
2/2

Setup:

Attach classic arm springs slightly above shoulder-height. Select the distance so that the exercise can be performed completely without any evasive movements. Usually it is closer than for the Boxing exercise, and the springs often hang through at the beginning. Standing in a small V outside the Cadillac, looking away from it. The hands hold the handles, the fingers are stretched. Bend the arms and move both hands to the right and left side of the face.

Purpose of the Exercise:

Strengthening of the pectoralis major, deltoideus, triceps brachii, serratus anterior, infraspinatus and biceps. Stabilization of the abdominal muscles. Fully body tension.

Execution: 3x -6x per side

Lunge with the right leg. Then stretch the arms upward parallel and diagonally. Viewed from the side there is an imaginary line from the left heel to the left hand.
Move the stretched arms downward in front of the hip. Turn the palms of the hands toward each other as much as necessary to evade the loops or aluminium bows of the handles with the back of the hands.
Raise the arms back up until the imaginary diagonal from the heels to the fingertips is reached again.
With a step backward, bring both feet together in the small "V" and move the hands next to the face with the elbows at shoulder level.

Switch legs.

Common Mistakes:

The distance was chosen incorrectly and the body loses its stability during the exercise.
The stability of the scapulae is given up and they constantly move. There is often an excessive protraction of the scapulae during the forward movement of the arms.
The arms are not fully stretched.

Modifications or Variations:

In the lunge position, perform three large arm circles through the full range of motion of the shoulder joint. Then change direction. The same sequence after changing legs.

Contraindications/Risks: -

21. Arm Circles Standing (T)
1/3

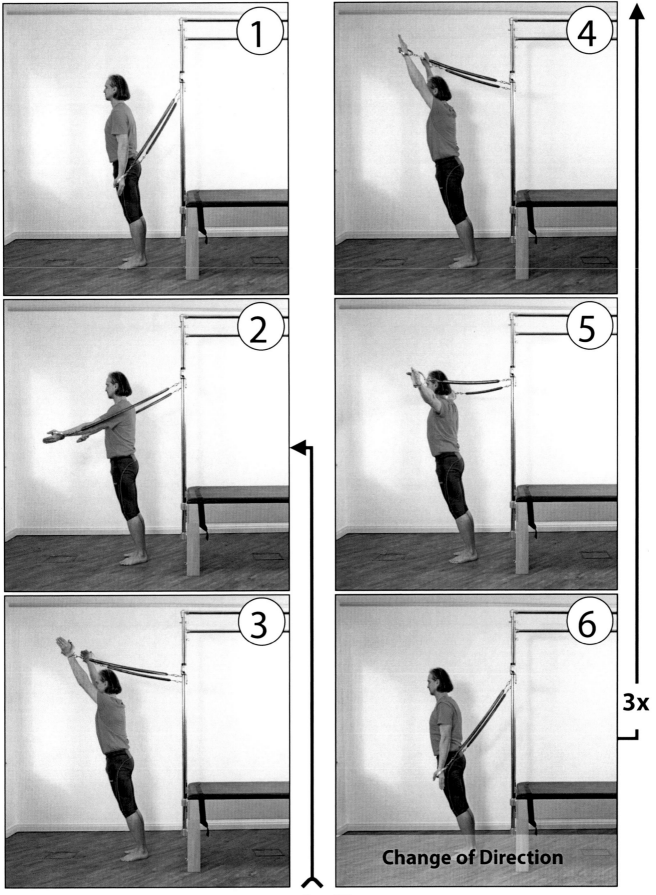

Change of Direction

3x

21. Arm Circles Standing (T)
2/3

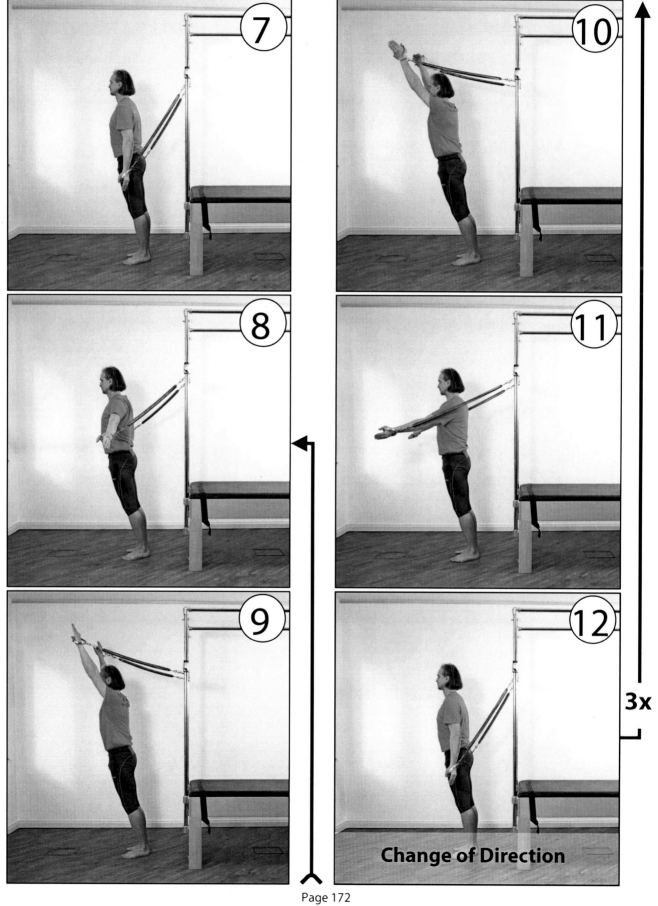

Change of Direction

3x

21. Arm Circles Standing (T)
3/3

Setup:

Attach classic arm springs slightly above shoulder-height. Select the distance so that the exercise can be performed completely without any evasive movements. Standing in a small V outside the Cadillac, looking away from it. The hands hold the handles, the fingers are stretched. The arms are at the sides of the body. The palms of the hands face forward.

Purpose of the Exercise:

Increasing the motion radius of the shoulders.
Stabilization of the shoulders.
Strengthening of the deltoid, pectoralis major, infraspinatus, triceps and biceps.

Execution: 5x per side

Direction 1: Raise the arms together, <u>with the palms first facing forward, then upward on shoulder-height and forward again when stretched up all the way.</u> Now bring the arms to the sides of the body and then downward, next to the hips. Make the circles as large as possible. Viewed from the front, the circles are half-circles, as the movement through the "center" is performed in a straight line with the arms parallel.
Repeat 3x - 5x, then change the direction.

Direction 2: Raise the arms up, sideward of the body, with <u>the palms continuously facing forward</u>. When stretched all the way up, rotate the arms as much as possible, so that they point backward. While lowering them in front of the body, <u>the palms face upward on shoulder-height and forward when brought all the way down.</u>
Repeat 3x - 5x.

Common Mistakes:

Already in the starting phase, the shoulders round forward.
When the arms point upward, the shoulders are raised along with them.

Modifications or Variations:

In case of preexisting shoulder problems, only perform the exercise up until shoulder-height.
Instead of the small V use a lunge position.

Contraindications/Risks:

The position of the arms above the head is too demanding for the shoulder and should not be performed in case of shoulder problems.

22. Triceps Push Out (T)
1/2

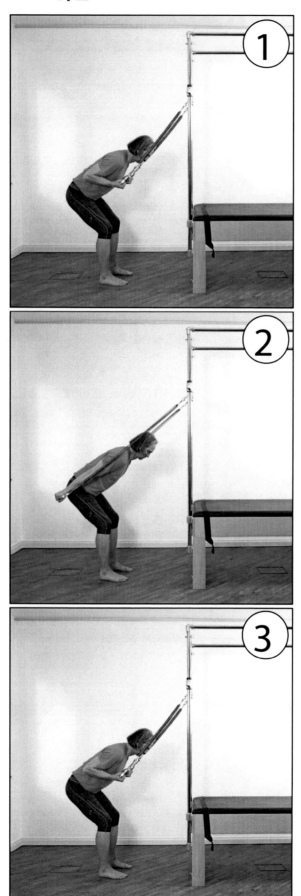

22. Triceps Push Out (T)
2/2

Setup:

Attach arm springs slightly above shoulder-height. Select the distance and the springs so that the exercise can be performed completely without any evasive movements.

Standing with the feet parallel and hip-wide apart outside Cadillac, looking toward it. Bent legs. The upper body is stretched and leaned forward. The head forms one line with the torso. The hands hold the handles and form fists. The arms are bent. The upper arms press against the torso.

Purpose of the Exercise:

Strengthening of the latissimus dorsi, triceps and posterior part of the deltoid.
Stabilization of the entire trunk and leg musculature.

Execution: 5x - 10x per direction

Stretch the arms downward into a straight line, bringing them backward until they are as stretched as possible. Then bend them again.

After 5-10 repetitions change the direction.

Common Mistakes:

Bending the upper body too far forward, until it is almost parallel to the floor.
The elbows/upper arms lose the contact to the torso and are not moved closely next to the body.
The arms are never fully stretched.

Modifications or Variations: -

Contraindications/Risks: -

23. The Butterfly / The Bat (T)
1/3

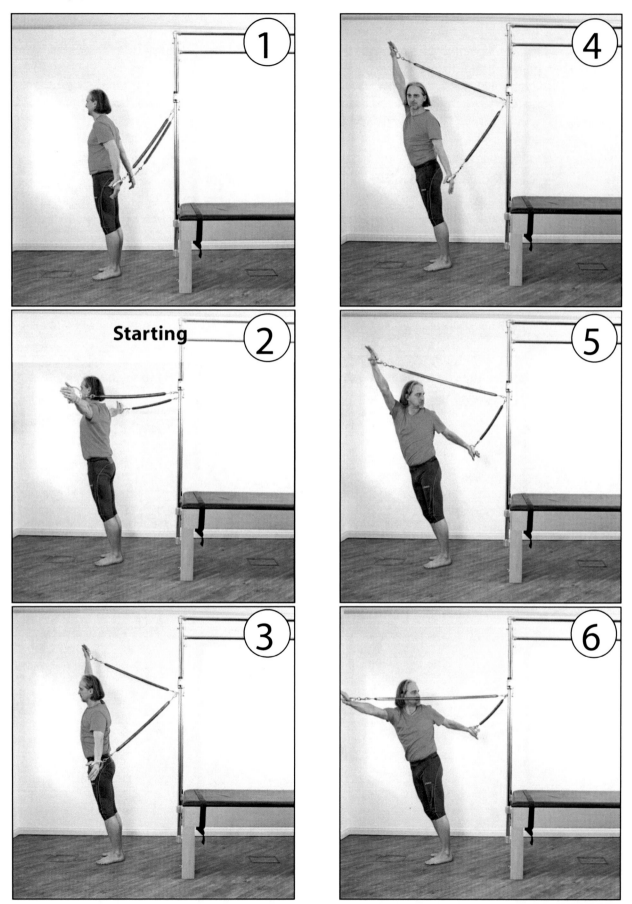

23. The Butterfly / The Bat (T)
2/3

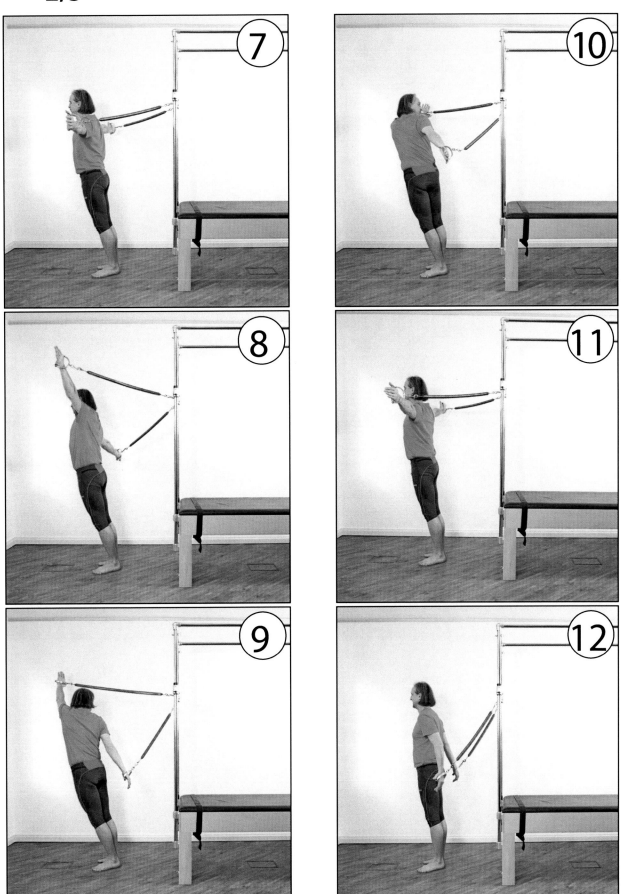

23. The Butterfly / The Bat (T)
3/3

Setup:

Attach arm springs slightly above shoulder-height. Select the distance and the springs so that the exercise can be performed completely without any evasive movements. Standing in a small V outside the Cadillac, looking away from it. The hands hold the handles, the fingers are stretched. The springs are not stretched yet but also do not hang loosely. Bring the arms up until slightly below shoulder-height, stretched to the sides.

Purpose of the Exercise:

Mobilization, particularly of the thoracic spine in the rotation with slight resistance.
Strengthening of the oblique abdominal muscles and the deltoid.
Coordinative training of the shoulder stabilizers.

Execution: 3 - 5 sets

Raise the right arm toward the ear and simultaneously lower the left arm toward the left side of the body with a slight lateral flexion to the left.
Starting from the chest, rotate to the left and follow the bending of the lateral flexion. The pelvis only follows once the upper body has reached the end of its range of motion. The upper body forms an arch. Keep the right arm close to the ear until the upper body has completed a 90 degree rotation. Only then, slowly lower the upper, right arm slightly below shoulder height and raise the lower, left arm to slightly below shoulder height. During the whole movement, try to maintain a slight tension in the springs.
Both arms move away from each other at one height like repulsing magnets, increasing the rotation of the upper body while in flexion. Looking backward, at the Cadillac.
Then rotate back the same way until both arms are in the same starting position as for the Hug.
Switch sides.

Raise the left arm toward the ear and simultaneously lower the right arm toward the right side of the body with a slight lateral flexion to the right.
Starting from the chest, rotate to the right and follow the bending of the lateral flexion. The pelvis only follows once the upper body has reached the end of its range of motion. The upper body forms an arch. Keep the upper, left arm close to the ear until the upper body has completed a 90 degree rotation. Only then, slowly lower it slightly below shoulder height and raise the lower, right arm to slightly below shoulder height. During the whole movement, try to maintain a slight tension in the springs.
Both arms move away from each other at one height like repulsing magnets, increasing the rotation of the upper body while in flexion. Looking backward, at the Cadillac.
Then rotate back the same way until both arms are in the same starting position as for the Hug.

Common Mistakes:

There is no lateral flexion at the beginning.
Giving up the bending during the exercise, causing the back to stretch.
The arms do not pull away from each other at the end of the exercise.
The arms are not at the same height in the end position, looking to the back.

Modifications or Variations: -

Contraindications/Risks: -

24. Full Butterfly / Full Bat (T)
1/4

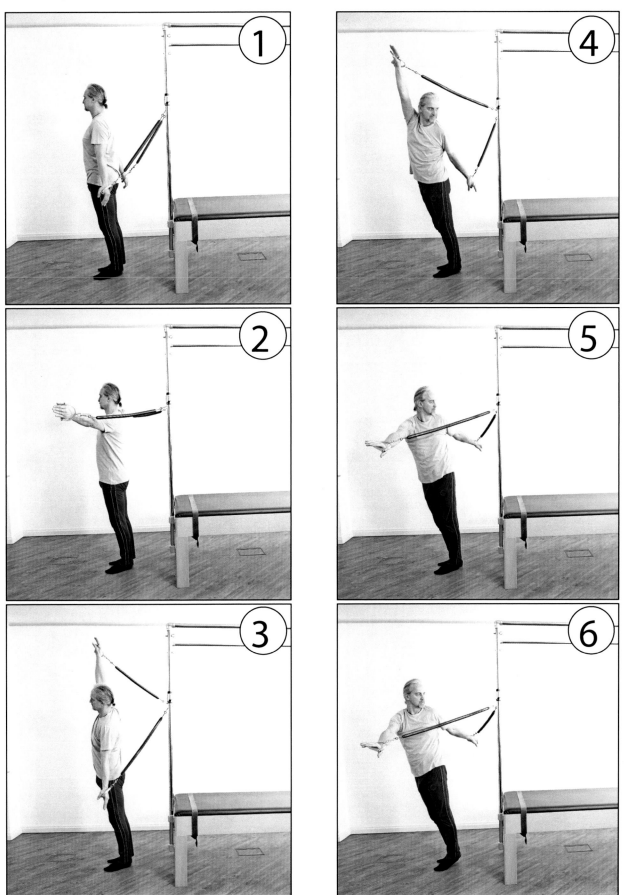

24. Full Butterfly / Full Bat (T)
2/4

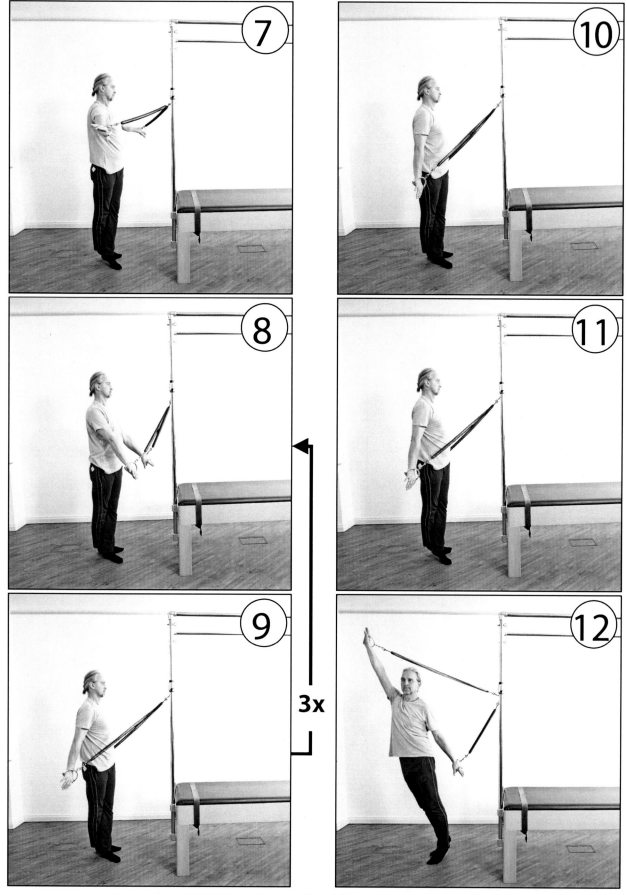

24. Full Butterfly / Full Bat (T)
3/4

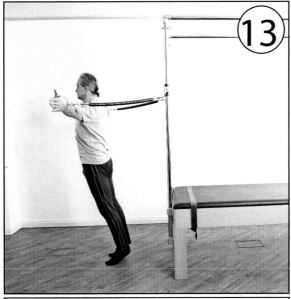

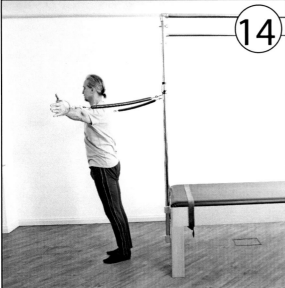

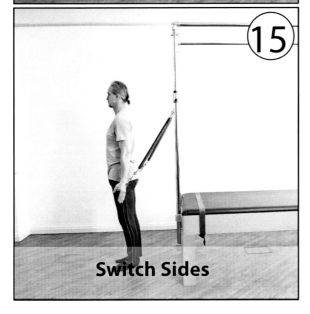

Switch Sides

Setup:
Attach arm springs slightly above shoulder-height. Select the distance and the springs so that the exercise can be performed completely without any evasive movements. Standing in a small V outside the Cadillac, looking away from it. The hands hold the handles, the fingers are stretched. The springs are not stretched yet but also do not hang loosely. Bring the arms up until slightly below shoulder-height, stretched to the sides.

Purpose of the Exercise:
Mobilization, particularly of the thoracic spine in the rotation with slight resistance.
Strengthening of the oblique abdominal muscles and the deltoid.
Coordinative and balance training.

24. Full Butterfly / Full Bat (T)
4/4

Execution: 3x - 5 sets

Raise the right arm toward the ear and simultaneously lower the left arm toward the left side of the body with a slight lateral flexion to the left.

Starting from the chest, rotate to the left and follow the bending of the lateral flexion. The pelvis only follows once the upper body has reached the end of its range of motion. The upper body forms an arch. Keep the right arm close to the ear until the upper body has completed a 90 degree rotation. Only then, slowly lower it slightly below shoulder height and raise the lower, left arm to slightly below shoulder height. During the whole movement, try to maintain a slight tension in the springs.

Both arms move away from each other at one height like repulsing magnets, increasing the rotation of the upper body while in flexion. Looking backward, at the Cadillac. Come up onto both the tiptoes and balls of the feet, and let the feet rotate until the body faces the Cadillac. Lower the heels and move the arms to the sides of the body. Pull them back 3x, closely past the body.

Then come up onto the tiptoes and balls of the feet again, raise the arms and rotate back the same way until both arms are in the same starting position as for the Hug. Lower the heels again.

Switch sides.

Raise the left arm toward the ear and simultaneously lower the right arm toward the right side of the body with a slight lateral flexion to the right.

Starting from the chest, rotate to the right and follow the bending of the lateral flexion. The pelvis only follows once the upper body has reached the end of its range of motion. The upper body forms an arch. Keep the left arm close to the ear until the upper body has completed a 90 degree rotation. Only then, slowly lower it slightly below shoulder height and raise the lower, right arm to slightly below shoulder height. During the whole movement, try to maintain a slight tension in the springs.

Both arms move away from each other at one height like repulsing magnets, increasing the rotation of the upper body while in flexion. Looking backward, at the Cadillac. Come up onto both the tiptoes and balls of the feet, and let the feet rotate until the body faces the Cadillac. Lower the heels and move the arms to the sides of the body. Pull them back 3x, closely past the body.

Then come up onto the tiptoes and balls of the feet again, raise the arms and rotate back the same way until both arms are in the same starting position as for the Hug. Lower the heels again.

Common Mistakes:

There is no lateral flexion at the beginning.
The arms do not pull away from each other at the end of the exercise.
The arms are not at the same height in the end position, looking to the back.

Modifications or Variations: -

Contraindications/Risks: -

Preliminary remarks for the Rowing series

The Rowing series is traditionally performed on the Reformer and consists of six exercises that are usually performed in a series:

- Rowing Back 1 - Into the Sternum

- Rowing Back 2 - 90 Degrees

- Rowing Front 1 - From the Chest

- Rowing Front 2 - From the Hips

- Shaving

- Hug

The series is traditionally performed at the beginning of the Reformer workout, after the Footwork, Hundred, Overhead and Coordination. It is integrated into the Advanced Reformer sequence and omitted during Basic or Intermediate. This shows clearly that the series is demanding in many ways.

The first four exercises in the series are among the most challenging in terms of coordination in Pilates and can be particularly demanding for the shoulder region.

The Rowing series was presumably not performed on the Cadillac by Joseph Pilates himself. Instead, as some Pilates teachers report, it was Romana Kryzanowska who brought many of the Reformer exercises to the Cadillac.

The series of exercises on the Cadillac feels completely different than on the Reformer and the flow of the exercises is not given in the same way. The exercises with the back facing the spring attachments in particular are often either too difficult or too simple on the Cadillac. It is not easy to find the right distance. For one-to-one training, we therefore recommend performing the Rowing series on the Reformer. For group classes on the Tower the Rowing Series can be a good addition.

25. Rowing - Into the Sternum (T)
1/3

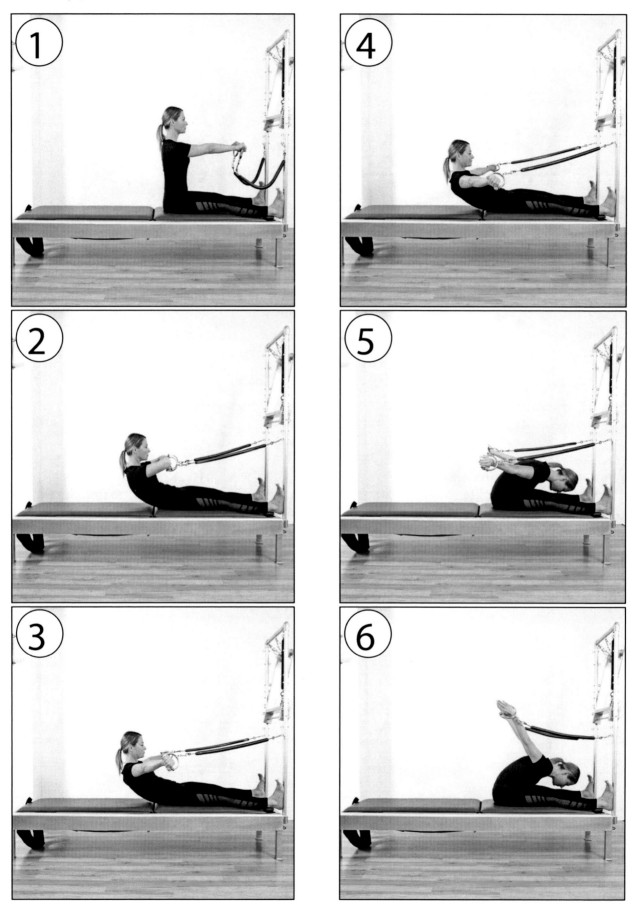

25. Rowing - Into the Sternum (T)
2/3

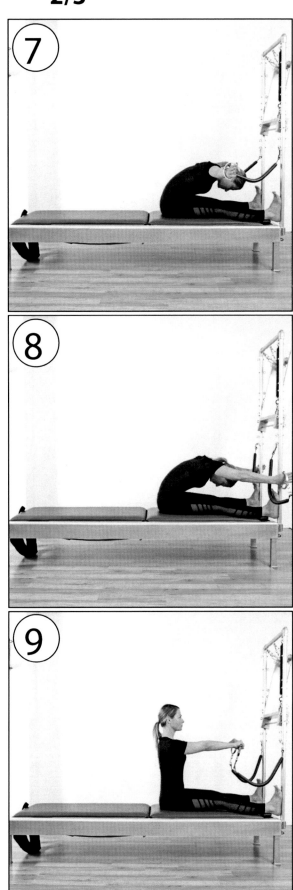

25. Rowing - Into the Sternum (T)
3/3

Setup:
Select the springs so that the exercise can be performed completely and without any evasive movements. *Attach arm springs at a height of 55 cm / 21 inches.* Sitting with the feet and heels against the vertical bars of the Cadillac frame. The arms are stretched forward, parallel to the mat. The palms face downward. Activate the sitting position by moving the ischial tuberosities inwardly toward each other and pulling the abdomen inward and upward.

Purpose of the Exercise:
Strengthening of the abdominal muscles.
Strengthening, particularly of the posterior shoulder musculature.
Stretch of the chest, shoulder and back musculature.

Execution: 3x
Bend the arms, move the elbows outward and bring the knuckles of the fingers of both hands against each other. The forearms rotate inward, the palms of the hands point downward and forward and the thumbs point toward the heart. The handle and spring run downward. The hands are in front of the chest with approx. one hand-width distance.
Simultaneously, roll back halfway (maximally up until the lumbar vertebrae) onto the mat, starting with the pelvis, and do not change the hand position in front of the chest. The upper chest and head remain upright. Stretch the arms to the sides, the palms pointing backward/downward.
Now pull the arms backward, maintaining the height (Image 4 to Image 5). Only then bend the body forward and bring the head toward the knees as far as possible. Pull the arms downward and backward (Image 6). If the shoulder flexibility is high, clasp the hands or make them touch. If the shoulder flexibility is low, leave the arms parallel.
Now, behind the body, raise the arms toward the ceiling as far as possible (Image 7). If the hands were clasped, first unclasp them. Turn the palms downward (thumbs pointing outward).
Now move your arms forward between the legs in a large curve. Usually the wrists have to rotate once to pass the vertical Cadillac poles. Already make sure that the handles are in the correct position (hanging down) for the start.
From there roll up again vertebra by vertebra, as if against a wall, and stretch the arms forward (palms pointing downward).

Common Mistakes:
Rolling too far down, all the way onto the thoracic spine.
The arms do not pull backward before the body is bent forward (Image 4-5).

Modifications or Variations:
The legs are parallel, instead of standing against the vertical poles.
Further modifications are already described above.
Traditionally, the palms of the hands are not yet rotated downward in the position with the arms stretched toward the ceiling (Image 7), but only on the way forward. However, this is a somewhat sub-optimal position for the shoulder and is therefore recommended differently here.

Contraindications/Risks:
The exercise is very demanding for the shoulder and can lead to shoulder problems if there are already pre-existing ones.
If the shoulder hurts during parts of the exercise, do not continue it. If parts of the exercise are pain-free, perform those parts and find a painless way to the starting position from there.

26. Rowing - 90 Degrees (T)
1/3

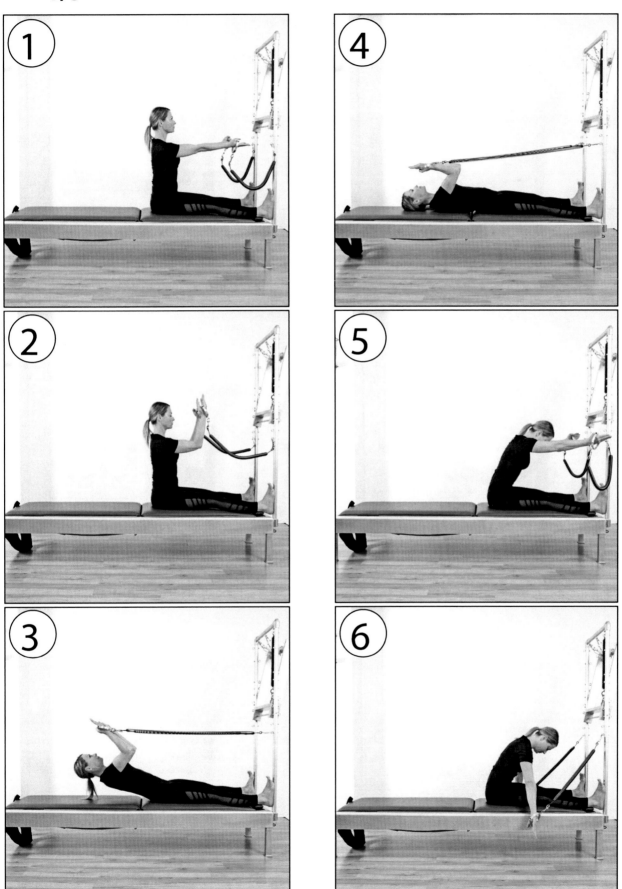

26. Rowing - 90 Degrees (T)
2/3

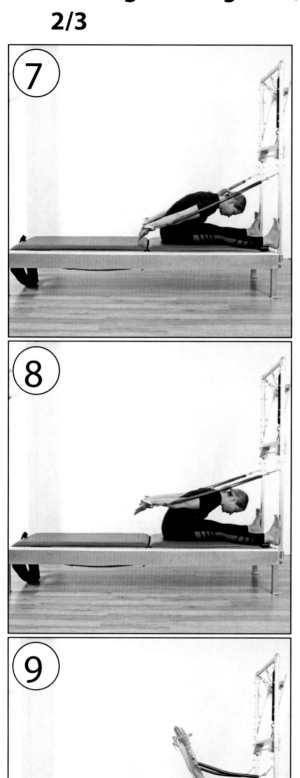

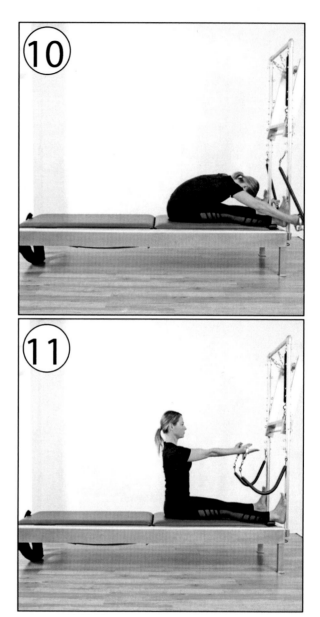

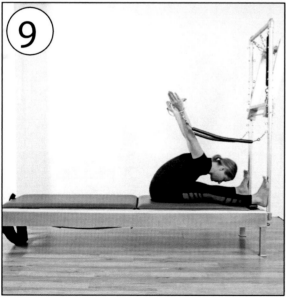

26. Rowing - 90 Degrees (T)
3/3

Setup:
Select the springs so that the exercise can be performed completely and without any evasive movements. *Attach arm springs at a height of 55 cm / 21 inches.* Sitting with the feet and heels against the vertical bars of the Cadillac frame. The arms are stretched forward, parallel to the mat. The palms face <u>upward</u>. Activate the sitting position by moving the ischial tuberosities inwardly toward each other and pulling the abdomen inward and upward.

Purpose of the Exercise:
Slight strengthening of the abdominal muscles.
Strengthening, particularly of the posterior shoulder musculature.
Stretch of the chest, shoulder and back musculature.

Execution: 3x
Bend the arms to slightly less than 90 degrees, keeping the elbows at shoulder-height.
<u>Only now</u> lean back with the back stretched and the arms in the same position. Keep looking forward for as long as possible. Fold back up in the same way and stretch the arms forward without lowering the elbows.
Bend forward and bring the head toward the knees as far as possible. Pull the arms past the Cadillac (Image 7) and downward, behind the body (Image 8). For a high shoulder flexibility, clasp the hands or make them touch. If the shoulder flexibility is low, keep the arms parallel.
Now, behind the body, raise the arms toward the ceiling as far as possible (Image 7). If the hands were clasped, first unclasp them. Turn the palms downward (thumbs pointing outward).
Now move your arms forward between the legs in a large curve. Usually the wrists have to rotate once to pass the vertical Cadillac poles. Already make sure that the handles are in the correct position (hanging down) for the start.
From there roll up again vertebra by vertebra, as if against a wall, and stretch the arms forward (palms pointing downward).

Common Mistakes:
The arms are bent too much and the work is brought from the posterior chain into the anterior chain of the chest muscles.
The arm position in relation to the upper body is changed during the backward leaning.
At the end of the exercise one hangs backward in the lumbar spine, while the thoracic spine is pushed forward too much to simulate a straight line (inverted lordosis).

Modifications or Variations:
The legs are parallel, instead of standing against the vertical poles.
Further modifications are already described above.
Traditionally, the palms of the hands are not already rotated downward in the position with the arms stretched toward the ceiling (Image 7), but only on the way forward. However, this is a somewhat sub-optimal position for the shoulder and is therefore recommended differently here.

Contraindications/Risks:
The exercise is very demanding for the shoulder and can lead to shoulder problems if there are already pre-existing ones.
If the shoulder hurts during parts of the exercise, do not continue it. If parts of the exercise are pain-free, perform those parts and find a painless way to the starting position from there.

27. Rowing - From the Chest (T)
1/2

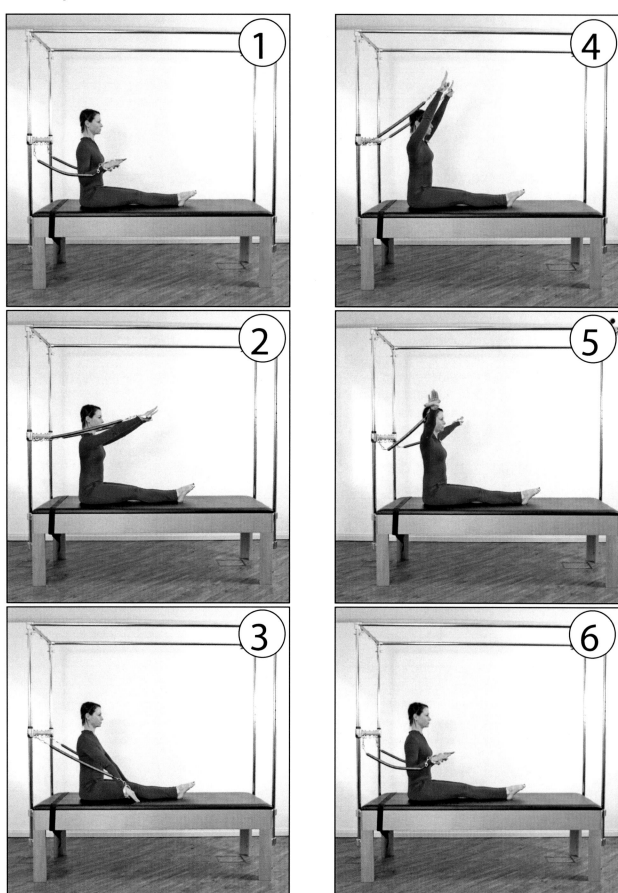

27. Rowing - From the Chest (T)
2/2

Setup:
Select the springs and distance so that the exercise can be performed completely and without any evasive movements. *Attach arm springs at a height of 55 cm / 21 inches.* Sitting with closed legs, looking away from the spring attachments, with the <u>feet in point position</u>. Bent elbows, the hands close to the chest, the forearms parallel to each other and the palms face downward. The springs come from above (exactly opposite to the exercise on the Reformer).

Activate the sitting position by moving the ischial tuberosities inwardly toward each other and pulling the abdomen inward and upward.

Purpose of the Exercise:
Increasing the motion radius of the shoulders.
Stabilization of the muscles, which move the shoulders.
Strengthening of the pectoralis major, deltoid, hip flexor and back extensor with the focus on the multifidus.
Slight strengthening of the latissimus dorsi when moving the arm from the top down to shoulder height.

Execution: 3x
Stretch the arms upward half diagonally without overstretching or locking them in place. Maintaining the upright sitting position, move the stretched arms downward to the mat and, from there, completely upward to the point where the shoulders are not yet raised. Move the arms outward and downward in a large curve. The hands point downward. The idea is to become taller as the arms move to the side.
When the hands are approximately in the starting position, bend the arms again and return to the starting position.

Common Mistakes:
The arms are not fully stretched.
The arms are overstretched or locked in place.
While lowering the arms, the upper body bends forward.
During the downward movement from the very top to the front (Image 4 to Image 5), the palms point forward instead of downward.

Modifications or Variations:
In case of preexisting shoulder problems, only perform the exercise up until shoulder-height.

Contraindications/Risks:
The overhead position of the arms is very demanding for the shoulder and should not be performed in case of shoulder problems.

28. Rowing - From the Hip (T)
1/3

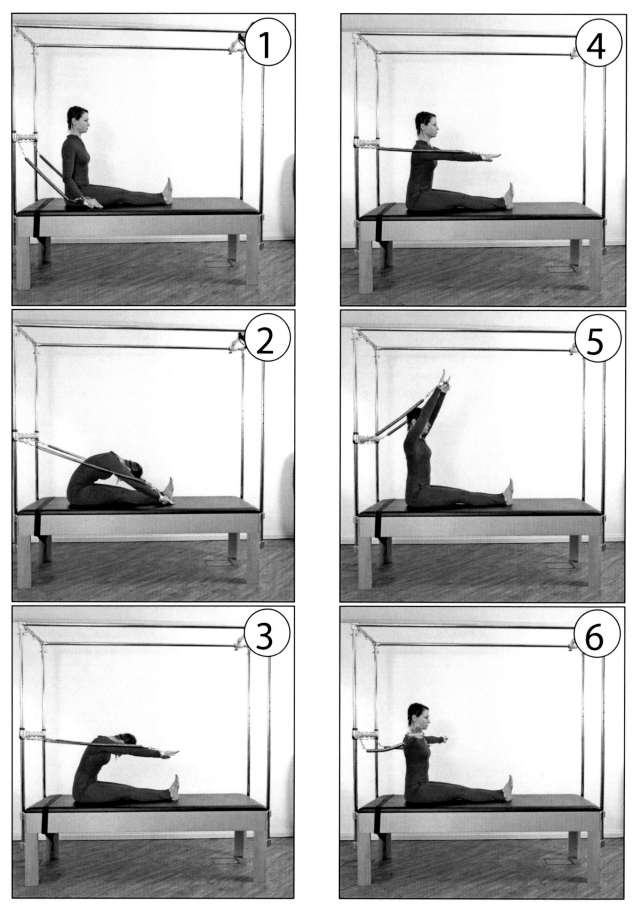

28. Rowing - From the Hip (T)
2/3

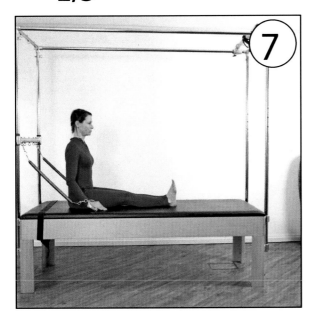

28. Rowing - From the Hip (T)
3/3

Setup:

Select the springs and distance so that the exercise can be performed completely and without any evasive movements. *Attach arm springs at a height of 55 cm / 21 inches.* Sitting with closed legs, looking away from the spring attachments, <u>with the feet flexed</u>. Place the hands on the mat, next to the hip, pointing <u>downward</u>. The springs come from above (exactly opposite to the exercise on the Reformer).

Activate the sitting position by moving the ischial tuberosities inwardly toward each other and pulling the abdomen inward and upward.

Purpose of the Exercise:

Stretch of the leg backs and the back muscles.
Increasing the motion radius of the shoulders.
Stabilization of the muscles, which move the shoulders.
Strengthening of the abdominal muscles, hip flexors, back extensors and the deltoid.
Slight strengthening of the latissimus dorsi when moving the arm from the top down to shoulder height.

Execution: 3x

Slide forward along the outer leg sides as far as possible with the palms on the mat. From the end position, slowly roll up the back from below as if against an invisible wall. The arms are parallel to the mat. From there, come all the way up to the point where the shoulders are not yet raised. Move the arms outward and downward in a large curve. The hands point downward. The idea is to become taller as the arms move to the sides.

When the hands are approximately at the height of the starting position, bend the arms again and return to the starting position.

Common Mistakes:

The arms are not fully stretched.
The arms are overstretched or locked in place.
The flexion of the feet or the stretching of the legs is given up when the hands are pushed forward.
The torso is partly brought back stretched, instead of vertebra by vertebra.
During the downward movement from the very top to the front (Image 4 to Image 5) the palms point forward instead of downward.
At the end of the exercise one hangs backward in the lumbar spine, while the thoracic spine is pushed forward too much to simulate a straight line (inverted lordosis).

Modifications or Variations:

In case of preexisting shoulder problems, only perform the exercise up until shoulder-height.

Contraindications/Risks:

The overhead position of the arms is very demanding for the shoulder and should not be performed in case of shoulder problems.

29. Rowing - Shaving (T)
1/2

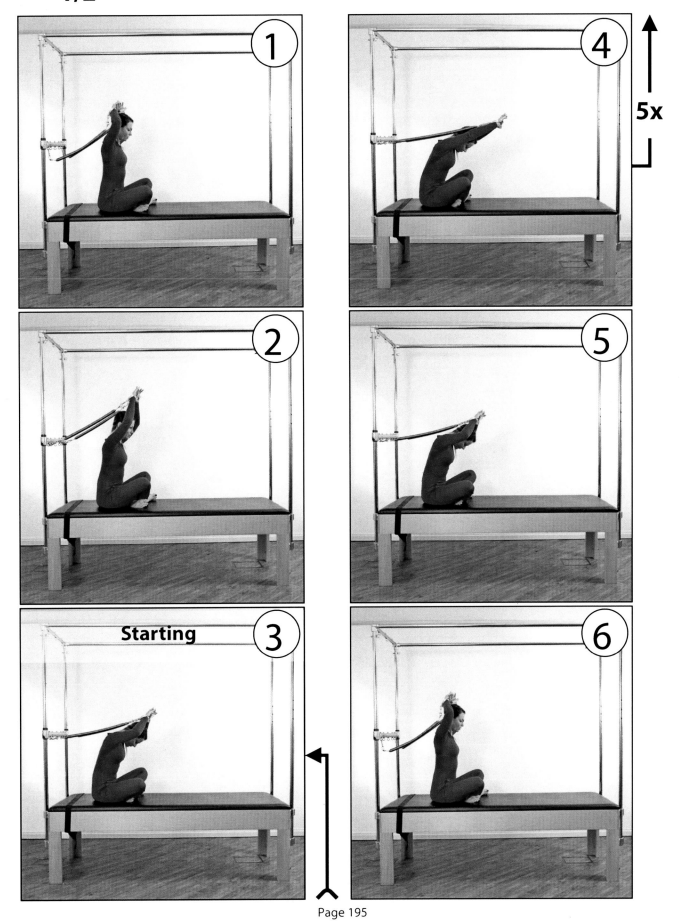

29. Rowing - Shaving (T)
2/2

Setup:

Select the springs and distance so that the exercise can be performed completely and without any evasive movements. *Attach arm springs at a height of 55 cm / 21 inches.* Sitting cross-legged, looking away from the spring attachments. The hands hold the handles with the palms facing forward. Bend the elbows outward and put the hands behind the head. Keep the elbows opened. Place the thumb of the right and left hand on top of each other as well as both index fingers. The thumbs and index fingers form a diamond. The fingers press firmly against each other.

Activate the sitting position by moving the ischial tuberosities inwardly toward each other and pulling the abdomen inward and upward. Round the upper back forward halfway.

Purpose of the Exercise:

Stabilization of the shoulders and torso.
Strengthening of the triceps and deltoid through stabilization by the anterior serratus.

Execution: 5x

Move the hands upward diagonally from behind the head along an imaginary, straight line. The more the back is rounded, the more parallel to the floor the movement of the hands becomes, and the muscular focus of the exercise changes. In the half-diagonal position there is more torso work, while there is more spring force and less torso work with the arms parallel to the Cadillac mat, because the body weight can be used. Focus on shoulder stability and triceps.
Choose the angle according to the individual abilities.

After the last repetition, bring the arms back behind the head from above and change the seat to a cross-legged position. Transition to Hug.

Common Mistakes:

The rounding is given up due to a lack of required strength.
The head hangs down.
The shoulders lose their stability and move up toward the ears.
The thumbs or fingers lose contact.

Modifications or Variations: -

Contraindications/Risks:

The overhead position of the arms is very demanding for the shoulder and should not be performed in case of shoulder problems.

30. Rowing - Hug (T)
1/2

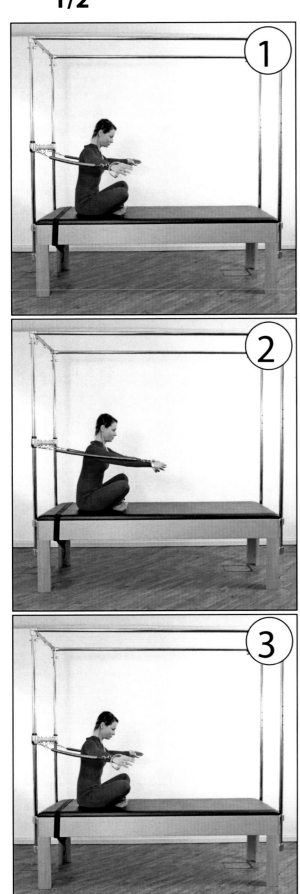

30. Rowing - Hug (T)
2/2

Setup:
Select the springs and distance so that the exercise can be performed completely and without any evasive movements. *Attach arm springs at a height of 55 cm / 21 inches.* Sitting cross-legged, looking away from the spring attachments. The hands hold the handles with forward-facing palms. The arms are opened and closely in front of the body. The elbows are smooth and not tensed. Activate the sitting position by moving the ischial tuberosities inwardly toward each other and pulling the abdomen inward and upward. Round the upper back forward halfway.

Purpose of the Exercise:
Breathing exercise.
Stabilization of the shoulders and torso.
Strengthening of the pectoralis major.

Execution: 3x - 6x
Move the arms in front of the body and simultaneously inhale. The chest is widened. The hands touch at the fingertips. Then exhale and bring the arms back toward the sides. The ribs sink downward. Bring the arms backward only until they are in front of the body. Repeat 3x.

Then move the arms in front of the body and simultaneously exhale. Try to wring all the air out of the lungs. The hands touch at the fingertips before inhaling and moving the arms to the sides again. Bring the arms backward only until they are in front of the body. Repeat 3x.

Common Mistakes:
The arms are moved behind the body.
The shoulders round as the arms are moved forward, the chest sinks in and the stability of the scapulae is given up.
The tightening of the ribs through the external abdominal muscles is lost as the arms are moved back to the sides.
The torso loses its upright position.

Modifications or Variations:
In case the shoulders are rounded forward, move the arms toward each other only until shoulder width.
To train different parts of the pectoralis major: The hands point slightly downward. During the movement in front of the body, the thumbs meet first. During the second repetition, the index fingers and so on, until the little fingers touch. On the way from the thumbs to the little fingers, the hands and forearms turn with every repetition until the hands are slightly upward facing. Then invert the movement and work back until the thumbs touch.
To train concentration and body awareness, perform the variation from above with closed eyes.

Contraindications/Risks: -

31. Teaser (M)
1/2

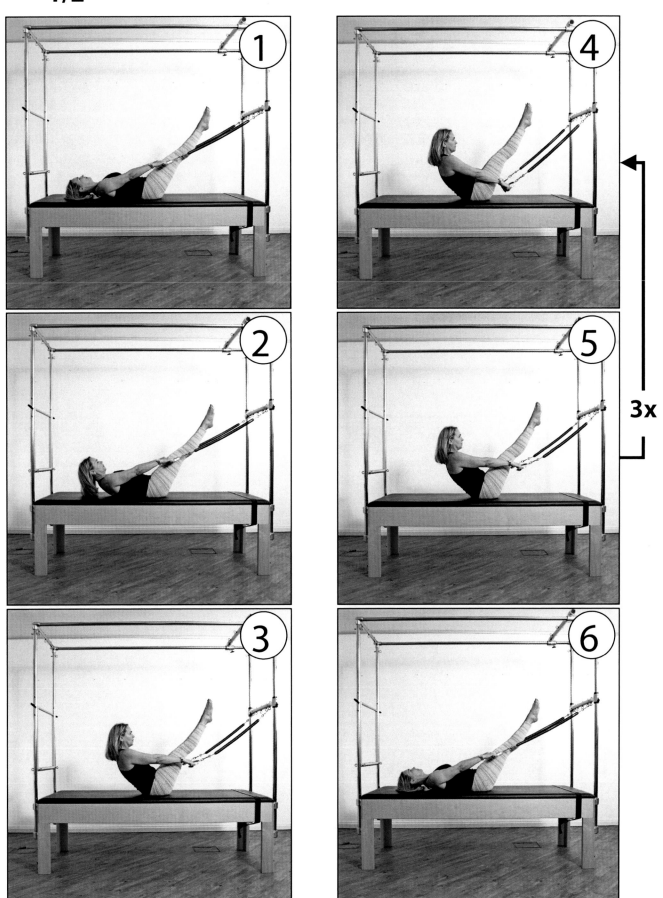

31. Teaser (M)
2/2

Setup:

Attach arm springs at approx. 80 - 85 cm / 31.5 - 33.5 inches, where, traditionally, leg springs are attached. Select the springs, spring attachment and distance so that the exercise can be performed completely and without any evasive movements. In this exercise, the optimal distance is even more important than usually and determines whether the exercise is performable at all, as well as whether the spring makes any difference or hangs down meaninglessly.

Lying, looking toward the spring attachments. The hands hold the handles with the palms facing downward. Pull the abdomen inward and upward and pull the knees toward the buttocks, stretch the legs upward and then slowly lower the legs to the personally achievable Teaser height. If possible, at 45 degrees.

Purpose of the Exercise:

Strengthening of the hip flexors and the entire abdominal musculature.

Execution: 3x - 5x

Lift the head and roll up into the Teaser while inhaling.
The lumbar spine remains round to prevent any unnecessary strain on the lumbar vertebrae.
Having reached the Teaser seat, press down the arms 3 times toward the Cadillac mat.
Roll back down vertebra by vertebra while keeping the legs at 45 degrees.
Repeat 3x - 5x.

Common Mistakes:

The arms are already pressed down during the roll-up movement.
The legs move up or down during the roll-up and roll-down movement.
The legs lose their inner tension.

Modifications or Variations: -

Contraindications/Risks: -

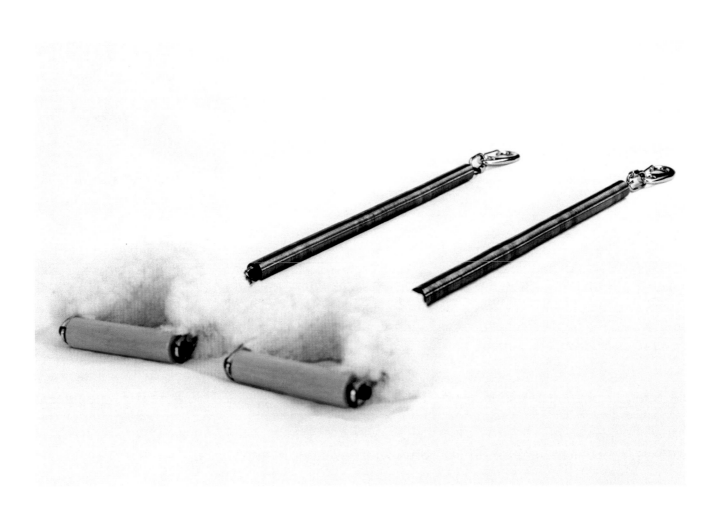

Baby/Arm Chair Springs

Preliminary remarks for the Baby/Arm Chair springs

The Pilates Arm Chair is a rare apparatus, only to be found in a few well equipped Pilates studios. Written knowledge about the Arm Chair is still rare to this day. The only first-hand source of information about the Arm Chair comes from MeJo Wiggin, who learned it directly from Romana Kryzanowska. Actually my training manual published in September 2016, inspired by the work of MeJo Wiggin was the first one to make this information available in writing.

The Pilates Arm Chair is especially suited for people with neck, shoulder issues, as well as working with students with kyphosis, scoliosis and osteoporosis.

If you don't have an Arm Chair, but a set of light springs such as, for example, Gratz Small Arm Chair Springs (also called Baby Springs) you can perform a whole range of Baby/Arm Chair exercises on the Cadillac with the help of a Reformer-Box.

Unfortunately, there are some special features of the Arm Chairs that are not available, such as the backrest, which slightly leans backward to give feedback regarding the shoulder position and support. In addition, the backrest of the classic Arm Chair is movable and goes forward and backward along with the movement of the practitioner. Hence, if the center of gravity is shifted forward, the springs and the backrest follow, so that the strength of the springs increases less in comparison to a non-movable spring attachment.

Therefore, Baby/Arm Spring exercises on the Cadillac are different on the Arm Chair even when using the same springs and will not be as effective. I have labeled the exercises still with a (T) for traditional because these are the same exercises, although it is clearly not traditional to do these exercises on the Cadillac with a Reformer Box. In my experience it is still a worthwhile option when working with clients with weak shoulders and arms e.g. in a group setting without an Arm Chair.

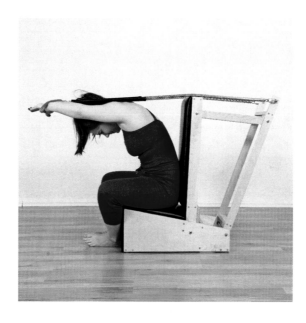

The most common positions during the Baby/Arm Spring exercises

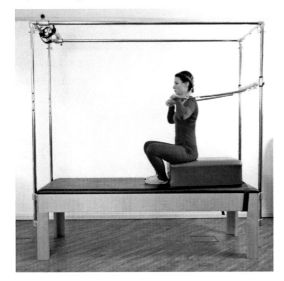

Sitting at the front edge of the Box

Sitting with a naturally straight spine. Legs in diamond shape, the soles of the feet press against each other. Pay attention to any dominance of one foot and correct it continuously. The heels are constantly pressing into the Reformer-Box. Both actions activate the insides of the legs. The position of the legs reminds of the leg position during the "Seal" on the mat. The position is well suited to open the lower back. If the position cannot be taken due to a lack of knee flexion, you can extend the front part of the Reformer-Box, for example through a thicker yoga block.

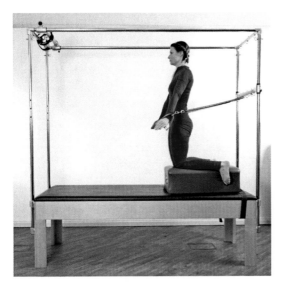

Kneeling with knees looking away from the spring attachments at the front edge of the Reformer-Box.

Take the rear feet a little higher sideways and press the inside of the feet into the Reformer-Box at the level of the metatarsophalangeal (MTP) joint. Then push the heels together gradually and without loosening the inner edges of the feet. The hip adductors and the gluteal muscles should be under tension. Straighten up.

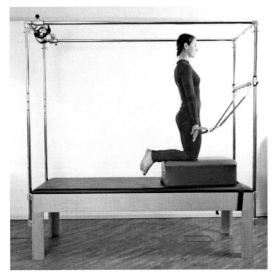

Kneeling in the direction of the spring attachments

Knees approximately in the center of the Reformer-Box, so that the feet and ankles have no contact with the Reformer-Box, the body is stretched up in a straight line from the knees upward. The thighs, knees and feet are closed and build up tension against each other (inner tension). The feet can be held either in dorsal flexion or plantar flexion.

1. Boxing (T)

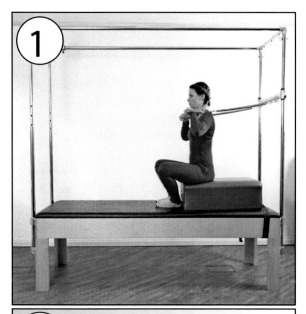

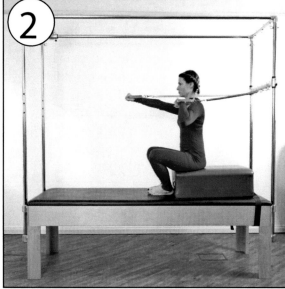

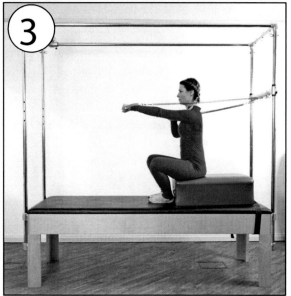

Setup:
Attach light arm springs slightly above shoulder height. Sitting on a Reformer-Box, with a straight back, legs in diamond shape. The hands hold the handles with the loops across the top of their wrists. The hands are at shoulder height. The elbows point outward.

Purpose of the Exercise:
Warming up the shoulders.
Stabilization of the shoulders.
Strengthening of the pectoralis major pars clavicularis and sternalis, anterior part of the deltoid muscle and triceps.

Execution: 5x -10x per side
One arm moves forward at, or slightly above, shoulder height. Box forward in line with, or slightly wider than, shoulder width but not less wide. While moving the arm backward, the other arm stretches forward. The pace is natural, not like a punch but not like slow motion either.

Common Mistakes:
The upper body turns along with the punch.
The shoulder blade of the moving arm loses its connection to the spine.

Modifications or Variations:
Place the legs in front of the Box or next to the Cadillac on Reformer-Boxes.

Contraindications/Risks: -

2. Small Arm Circles (T)

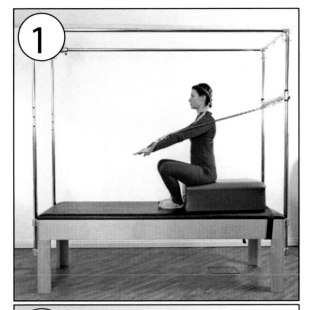

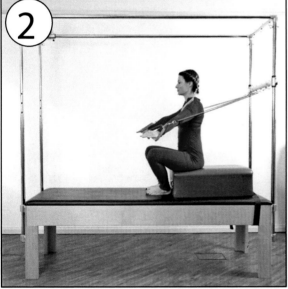

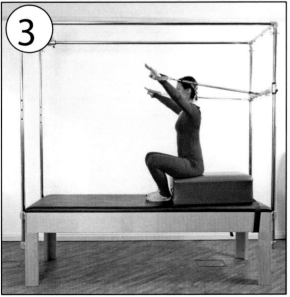

Setup:
Sitting on the Reformer Long Box, with a straight back, legs in diamond shape. The hands hold the handles with the loops across the top of the wrists. The hands are at shoulder height.

Purpose of the Exercise:
Warming up the shoulders.
Stabilization of the shoulders.
Coordinative training of the shoulder-stabilizing musculature.

Execution: 5x - 7x per side
At a little more than shoulder-width apart, stretch both arms forward, the palms facing the mat. First, lower the arms, then move them outward and then raise them toward shoulder height. Come back into the starting position. The palms constantly face the mat. Repeat five times, then change direction. Perform the circles large enough for the hands to always remain within the peripheral vision when looking straight ahead with the eyes. Although the exercise is called "Circles" they are actually rather semicircles, since the downward movement in the first direction is performed in a straight line.

Common Mistakes:
Already in the starting phase, the shoulders round forward.

Modifications or Variations:
In case of shoulder pain, perform smaller circles.
Place the legs in front of the Box or next to the Cadillac on Reformer Boxes.
If the springs or carabiners hurt on the forearms, turn the hands slightly (palms facing each other) and do not move them too close to each other.

Contraindications/Risks: -

3.   Hug (T)

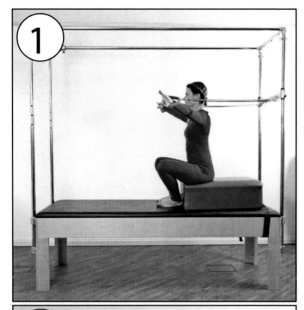

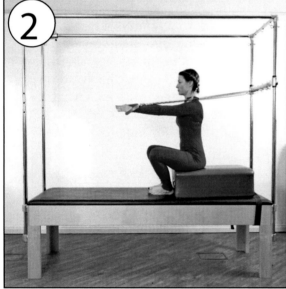

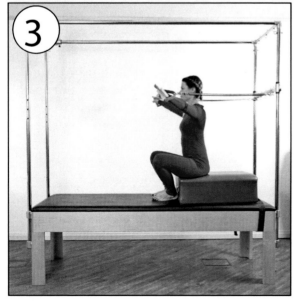

Setup:
Sitting on the Reformer Long Box, with a straight back, legs in diamond shape. The hands hold the handles with the loops across the top of the wrists. Both arms are opened outward, the hands still remain in front of the shoulders.

Purpose of the Exercise:
Strengthening of the pectoralis major.
Training of the muscles controlling the shoulder blades.

Execution: 5x
Bring the arms together in front of the body. The elbows are bent very slightly. The hands touch at the fingertips before the arms move back into the starting position.

Common Mistakes:
The shoulders round downward while moving the arms forward, the chest sinks down and the scapula stability is lost. The tension of the external abdominal muscles is lost, causing the ribs to wing, as the arms move back outward.

Modifications or Variations:
If the shoulders tend to round forward, move the arms together only until one reaches shoulder width.
Place the legs in front of the Box or next to the Cadillac on Reformer Boxes.
Use the exercise to train breathing: First, inhale when bringing the arms together and exhale while moving them outward. Repeat three times. Then exhale while bringing the arms together and let all the air out of the lungs. Inhale fully on the way back.
Concentration and coordination exercise: The small fingers of the left and right hand touch as they come to the center. During the next repetition, the ring fingers, then the middle fingers, etc. touch until the thumbs meet. The palms of the little fingers are turned upward. The closer one gets to the thumbs, the more the palms of the hands turn downward.

Contraindications/Risks: -

4. Hug with Chest Lift (T)

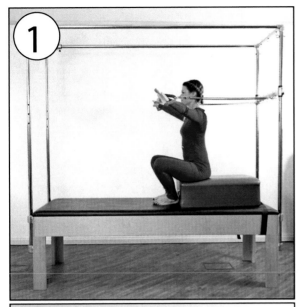

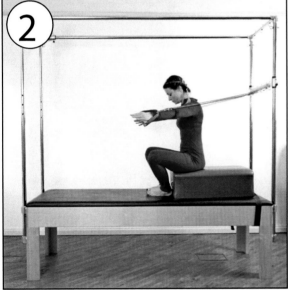

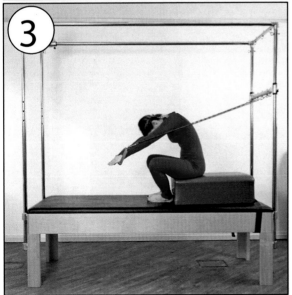

Setup:
Sitting on the Reformer Long Box with a straight back, legs in diamond shape.
The hands hold the handles with the loops across the top of the wrists. Both arms are opened outward, the hands still remain in front of the shoulders.

Purpose of the Exercise:
Stabilization of the shoulders despite flexion of the torso.
Strengthening of the pectoralis major and abdominal muscles.
Mobilization of the thoracic spine.

Execution: 5x
Move both arms forward. The elbows are bent very slightly. The hands touch at the fingertips.
At the same time, roll down until the thoracic spine is flexed. The lower back remains upright. While rolling back vertebra by vertebra, move the arms outward again.

Common Mistakes:
The "Chest Lift" part of the movement is performed too much by the head and not enough by "tilting" underneath the ribs.
Passive leaning against the springs instead of active work of the abdominal muscles.
The shoulders round when stretching the arms forward.
The tension of the external abdominal muscles is lost, causing the ribs to wing, while moving the arms outward again.

Modifications or Variations:
Place the legs in front of the Box or next to the Cadillac on Reformer Boxes.
If the shoulders tend to round toward the front, move the arms together only until shoulder width is reached.

Contraindications/Risks: -

5.   Kneeling Hug (T)

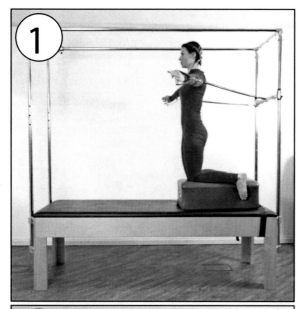

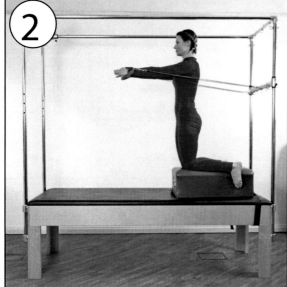

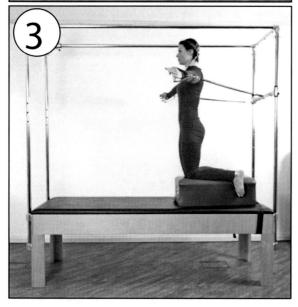

Setup:
Kneeling on the Reformer Long Box, with the feet at the side of the Box. Looking away from the spring attachments. Spring height below the scapulae. Both arms are opened to the sides, the hands still remain in front of the shoulders.

Purpose of the Exercise:
Stabilization of the shoulders and torso. Strengthening of the pectoralis major (higher spring tension in comparison to the prior seated Hug, which causes a higher training effect).

Execution: 5x
Move both arms forward. The elbows are bent very slightly. The hands touch at the fingertips before the arms move back into the starting position.

Common Mistakes:
The shoulders round while moving the arms forward, the chest sinks down and the scapula stability is lost. The tension of the external abdominal muscles is lost, causing the ribs to wing, while moving the arms outward again.

Modifications or Variations:
If the shoulders tend to round toward the front, move only the arms.

Contraindications/Risks: -

6.   Big Arm Circles (T)

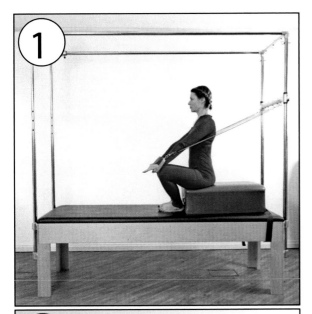

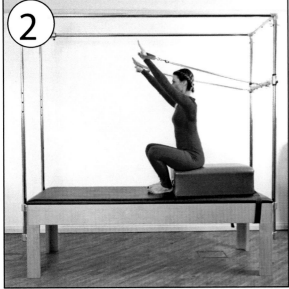

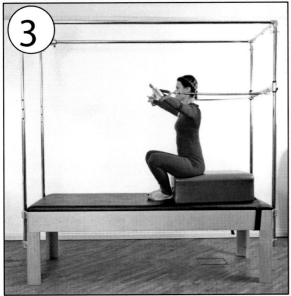

Setup:
Sitting on the Reformer Long Box with a straight back, legs in diamond shape. The hands hold the handles with the loops across the top of the wrists. The hands are at shoulder height.

Purpose of the Exercise:
Improving the range of motion in the shoulders. Stabilization of the muscles moving the shoulders. Strengthening of the pectoralis major and deltoid muscle. Slight strengthening of the latissimus dorsi when moving the arm from its uppermost position down to shoulder height.

Execution: 5x per side
Direction 1: Stretch the arms forward with the palms facing down. First, lower the arms and then move them outward. The palms constantly face down or forward when they are stretched up. Repeat five times, then change direction. Perform the circles as largely as possible.
Here, too, the circles are rather semicircles as the movement through the "center" is performed in a straight line.
Direction 2: Move the arms, with the palms facing forward, to the sides and then upward. Then, move the arms forward and, finally, downward pointing forward and down.

Common Mistakes:
The shoulders already round during the initial phase. When the arms point up, the shoulders are also lifted. The upper back is arched when the arms go further than 90 degrees.

Modifications or Variations:
Turning the hands at shoulder height so that the palms face up while lowering the arms during direction 1. Lifting the hands with the palms facing up (water scoop) during the opposite direction and turning the palms to face downward at shoulder height.
Place the legs in front of the Box or next to the Cadillac on Reformer-Boxes.

Contraindications/Risks: -

7. Kneeling Arm Circles (T)
1/2

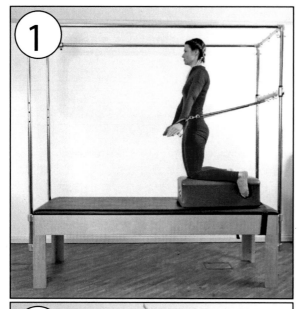

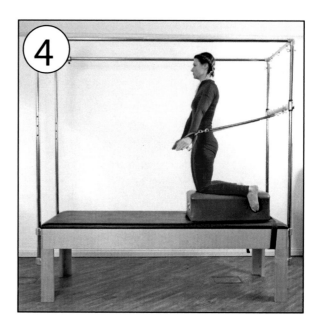

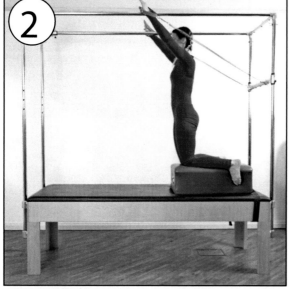

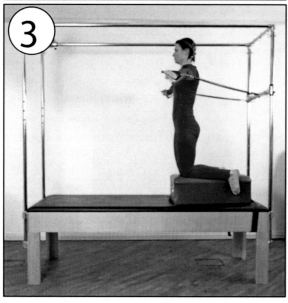

7. Kneeling Arm Circles (T)
2/2

Setup:
Kneeling on the Reformer Long Box with the feet at the sides of the Box. Looking away from the spring attachments. Spring height below the scapulae.

Purpose of the Exercise:
Improving the range of motion in the shoulders.
Stabilization of the shoulders and torso.
Strengthening of the deltoid muscle, pectoralis major, infraspinatus and biceps.

Execution: 5x per side
Direction 1: Raise both arms with the palms facing up. At the highest point, turn the palms to face forward. Move the arms to the sides and from there laterally toward the ground, the palms facing forward.
Repeat five times, then change the direction. Perform the circles as largely as possible.
Here, too, the circles are more like semicircles as the movement through the "center" is performed in a straight line.
Direction 2: Move the arms, with the palms facing forward, to the sides and then upward. Then, move the arms first forward and then down, pointing forward and down.

Common Mistakes:
The shoulders already round during the initial phase.
When the arms point up, the shoulders are also lifted.
Giving up the torso stability, too much tipping into the lordosis.

Modifications or Variations: -

Contraindications/Risks: -

8.   Sparklers (T)

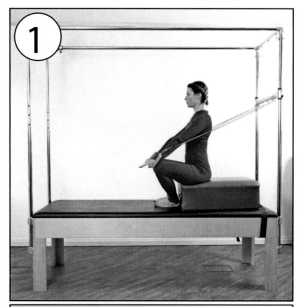

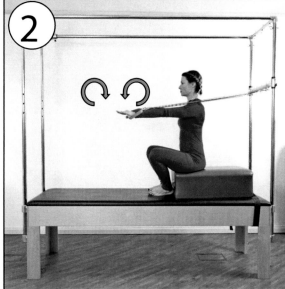

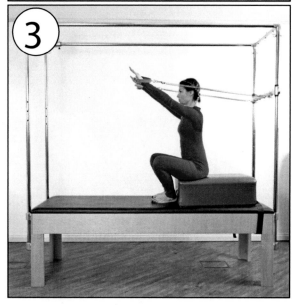

Setup:
Sitting on the Reformer Long Box with a straight back, legs in diamond shape. The hands hold the handles with the loops across the top of the wrists. The hands are at knee height.

Purpose of the Exercise:
Stabilization of the shoulders.
Coordinative training of the muscles stabilizing the shoulders.

Execution:
Perform small, quick circles as though drawing small circles of light with sparklers. Start slightly above thigh-height. While performing the small circles, move the arms upward until they cannot be raised any further without also raising the shoulders. Circle back down and then up again. Change the direction of the circles once you reach the top and circle back down, up and down again.

Common Mistakes:
The arms are not circled quickly and strongly enough.

Modifications or Variations:
The back is straight and leaned forward.
Place the legs in front of the Box or next to the Cadillac on Reformer Boxes.

Contraindications/Risks: -

9. Chest Expansion (T)

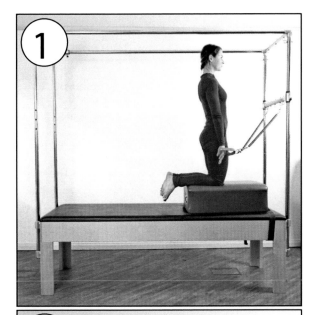

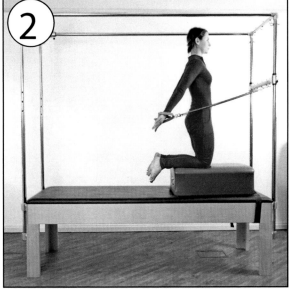

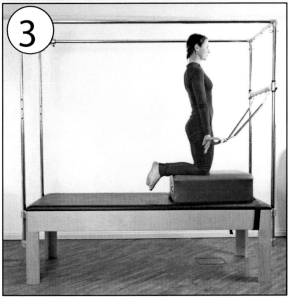

Setup:
Kneeling on the Reformer Long Box, looking toward the spring attachments, with the knees approximately in the center of the Reformer Box.

Purpose of the Exercise:
Strengthening of the latissimus dorsi, triceps and posterior part of the deltoid.
Slight stretch of the anterior deltoid.
Stabilization of the torso through a strengthening of the long back extensors and the gluteal muscles.
Training the mobility of the cervical and upper thoracic spine.

Execution: 5x
Bring the arms backward, sideways past the body. First, turn the head to the right, then to the left and then to the center. Only then move the arms back to the front until the springs are relaxed. Open the shoulders well throughout the movement and keep the torso upright. To optimize the rotation of the head, the shoulder adductors have to work and the shoulder abductors should be as relaxed as possible.

Common Mistakes:
The upper body sinks in and the shoulders are pulled forward, while the arms are rotated inward. In this case, turning the head is rather counterproductive.
The head is not rotated on one level, instead the chin is lowered during the rotation.

Modifications or Variations:
The arm is moved behind the body. From there, perform small pulses. Starts with 1 pulse and move the arm back completely, then 1, 2 pulses and move the arm back, then 1, 2, 3 pulses and back, then 1, 2, 3, 4 - and so on until the maximum of 10 pulses is reached. Then vice versa: 1,2,3,4,5,6,7,8,9 - and back. 1,2,3,4,5,6,7,8 - and back, and so on.

Contraindications/Risks: -

10. Kneeling Triceps Push up (T)

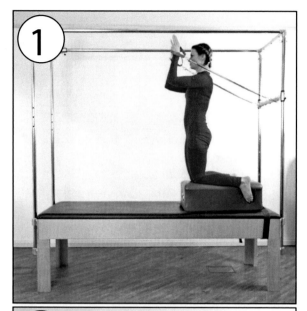

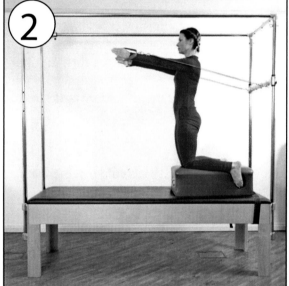

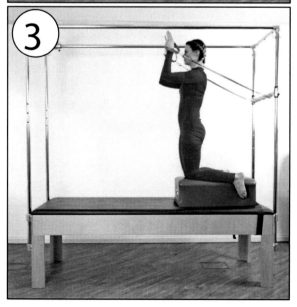

Setup:
Kneeling on the Reformer Long Box, with the feet at the sides of the Box. Looking away from the spring attachments. Spring height below the scapulae.

Purpose of the Exercise:
Strengthening of the triceps.
Stabilization of the torso and shoulders.

Execution: 3x - 7x
The outstretched arms are raised shoulder-wide apart. The palms face each other. Once the elbows are slightly above shoulder height, the elbows are bent and the forearms are moved back until a 90 degree angle is reached. Then stretch them out again. The elbows stay at the same height. Repeat this 4x.

Common Mistakes:
The elbows sink while bending the arms and are raised while extending the arms.
The shoulders are pulled up in a cramped way.
Giving up the torso stability, overly tilting into the lordosis.

Modifications or Variations:
Any seated position.

Contraindications/Risks: -

11. Long Arm Pull Back (M)

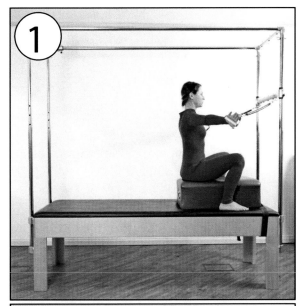

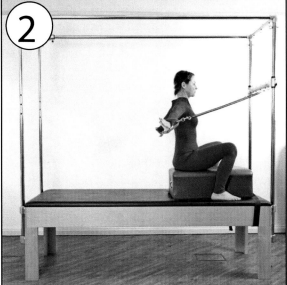

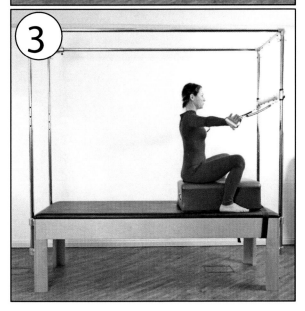

Setup:
Sitting on the Reformer Long Box, facing the spring attachments. Stretch the arms out to the sides at shoulder height. Turn the palms to face backward.

Purpose of the Exercise:
Strengthening of the posterior and center part of the deltoid muscle, the rhomboid muscle, triceps, teres major and subscapularis for the inner rotation at 90° abduction.

Execution: 3x sets with 5 pulses
Pull the arms backward until the springs are under tension and then perform small backward pulses.

Common Mistakes:
The chest is bent forward during the small pulses.

Modifications or Variations:
More difficult variation: Kneeling on the Box and looking away from the spring attachments.

Contraindications/Risks: -

12. One Arm Pull (M)

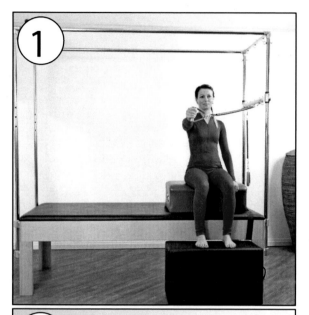

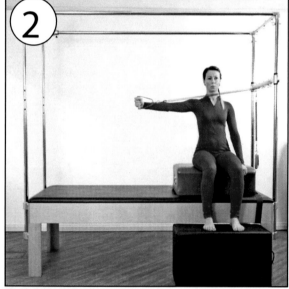

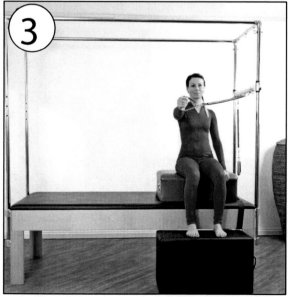

Setup:
Sitting sideways on a Reformer Box. Ideally, the feet should be placed on another Reformer Box. The outer arm should be stretched forward at shoulder level.

Purpose of the Exercise:
Strengthening of the posterior deltoid muscle. Stabilization of the serratus anterior, rhomboid muscle, lateral torso musculature and triceps.

Execution: 5x
Move the extended arm to the side in a large curve until it is in one line with the shoulders. Then bring it back slowly. This exercise is very similar to the first exercise of the Swakatee series "21. Swakatee (T)". However, the difference is that, in the One Arm Pull, the arm here is moved along the motion radius while stretched out, whereas the arm only slowly unfolds in Swakatee.

Common Mistakes:
The rhomboid muscles pull the scapulae back, causing the posterior deltoid muscle to be strengthened less.

Modifications or Variations:
Perform small pulses at the end of the movement.

Contraindications/Risks: -

13. Cross Arm Rotation (M)

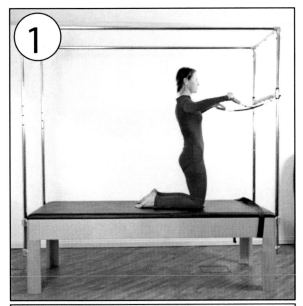

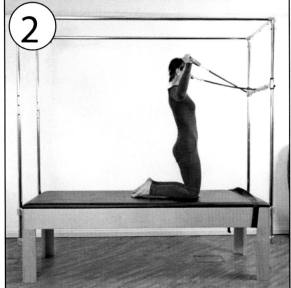

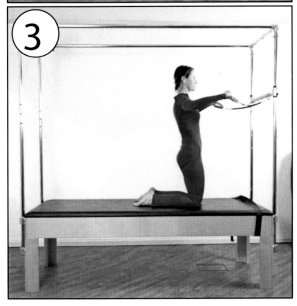

Setup:
Kneeling, looking toward the spring attachments. The springs cross while the hands/arms do not.

Purpose of the Exercise:
Strengthening of the infraspinatus, teres minor, posterior deltoid muscle and lower trapezius. Stabilization of the serratus anterior, central deltoid muscle and torso.

Execution: 5x
The elbows are at shoulder height. The upper arms form a long line with the shoulders. The forearms form a right angle to the upper arms. This way, the triceps has to work constantly. Imagine a rod running from one elbow to the other. The forearms rotate upward around this axis.

Common Mistakes:
The forearms fold inward and decrease the 90° angle. Giving up the stability of the torso, overly tilting into a lordosis.

Modifications or Variations:
If one side is weaker than the other, do additional repetitions with only this arm.

Contraindications/Risks: -

14. Shaving Straight Back (T)

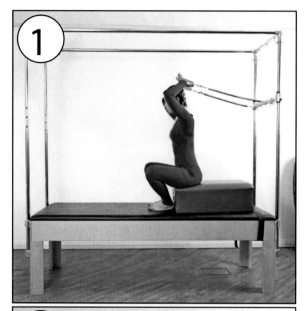

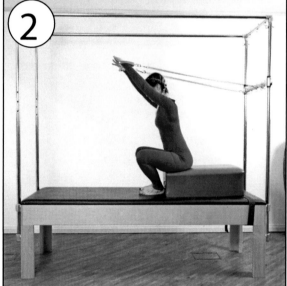

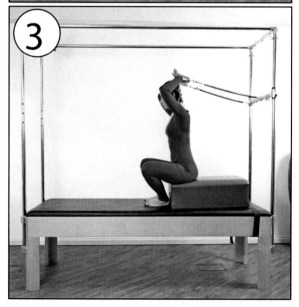

Setup:

Sitting, with a straight back and leaned forward. The legs are in diamond shape. The hands hold the handles with the loops across the top of the wrists. The thumbs and index fingers of both hands press against each other. The hands form a diamond and are held behind the neck. The elbows are wide.

Purpose of the Exercise:

Stabilization of the shoulders and torso. Strengthening of the triceps and deltoid muscle (higher spring tension than for Shaving Sitting Back), stabilized by the serratus anterior.

Execution: 5x

Move the hands up and down along an imaginary, diagonal line.

Common Mistakes:

The shoulders lose their stability and move up toward the ears.
The thumbs or fingers lose contact.

Modifications or Variations:

Place the legs in front of the Box or next to the Cadillac on Reformer Boxes.

Contraindications/Risks: -

15. Shaving Forward Round Back (T)

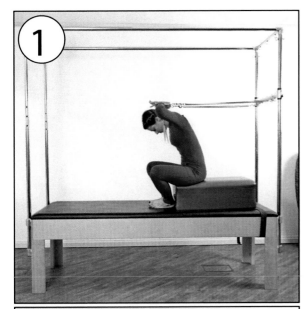

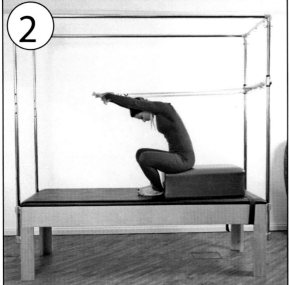

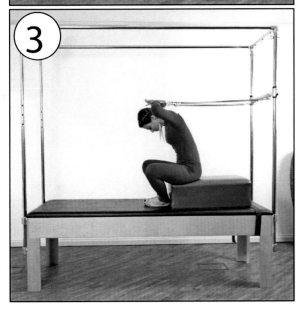

Setup:

Sitting, with a rounded back and bent forward. The hands hold the handles with the loops across the top of the wrists. The thumbs and index fingers of both hands press against each other. The hands form a diamond and are held behind the neck. The elbows are wide.

Purpose of the Exercise:

Stabilization of the shoulders.
Strengthening of the triceps and deltoid muscle (higher spring tension than for Shaving Straight Back), stabilized by the serratus anterior and all abdominal muscle groups.

Execution: 5x

Parallel to the ground, move the hands back and forth along an imaginary line.

Common Mistakes:

The shoulders lose their stability and move up toward the ears.
The thumbs or fingers lose contact.

Modifications or Variations:

Place the legs in front of the Box or next to the Cadillac on Reformer Boxes.

Contraindications/Risks: -

16. Chest Expansion and Extension (M)
1/2

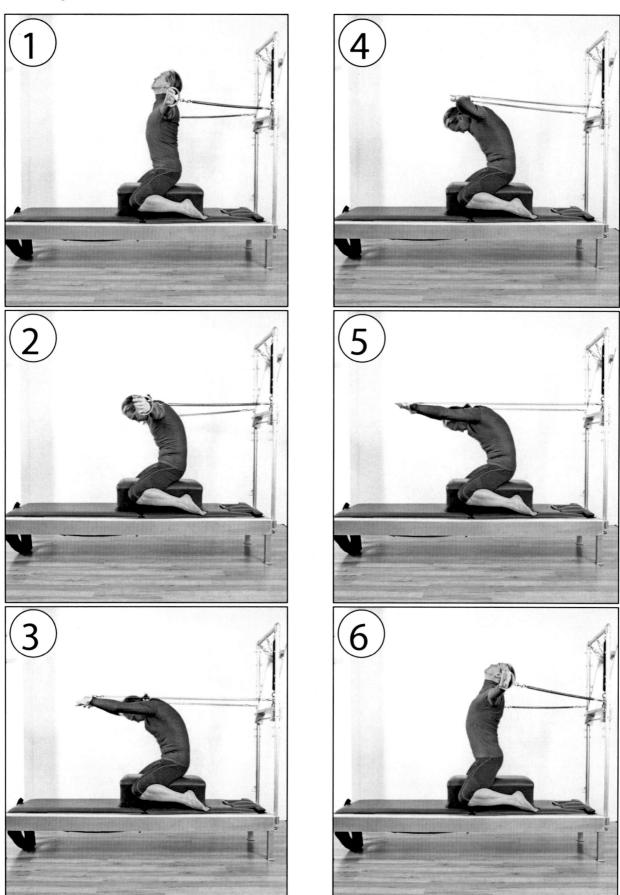

16. Chest Expansion and Extension (M)
2/2

Setup:
Sitting in the center of the Reformer Box, looking away from the spring attachments. The knees are opened and flexed. The feet point backward, a kind of heel seat with the Box between the legs. The handles are held by the hand. The arms are stretched out at shoulder height. Chest in extension.

Purpose of the Exercise:
Mobilisation of the spine by alternating between extension (arch) and flexion (curl).
Stabilization of the shoulders.
Strengthening of the triceps and deltoid with a stabilization by the serratus anterior, pectoralis major and all abdominal muscle groups.

Execution: 5x - 7x
Move the arms forward in a Hug while the upper body changes to a flexion in a "large C-curve". Looking down. The thumbs of both hands press strongly against each other, as do the index fingers. The hands form a diamond. Remaining in the C-curve, widen the elbows and move the hands back toward the neck. Move the hands forward again along an imaginary line, which is parallel to the floor, as in "Shaving Forward Round Back". Move the arms back to the sides, stretch the upper body and bring the chest into the extension.

Common Mistakes:
During the Hug the shoulders are rounded as the arms are moved forward, the chest sinks and the scapula stability is given up. The ribs are winged as the arms are moved back to the sides and the external abdominal muscles lose their stability.
During the shaving movement, the shoulders lose their stability and move toward the ears.

Modifications or Variations:
Place the legs in front of the Box or next to the Cadillac on Reformer Boxes.
Legs in a diamond, the soles of the feet are on top of each other.

Contraindications/Risks: -

17. Swimming Straight Back (M)

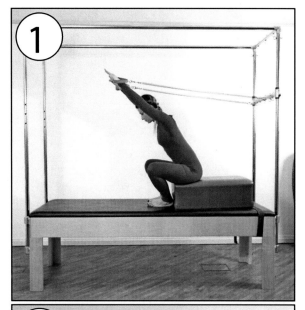

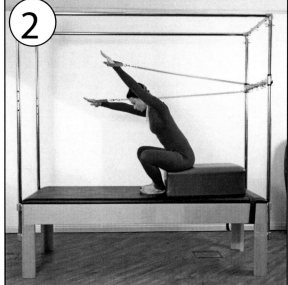

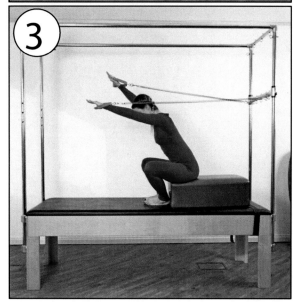

Setup:
Sitting, with a straight back and leaned forward. The hands hold the handles with the loops across the top of the wrists. The arms are stretched as an extension of the spine.

Purpose of the Exercise:
Mobilization of shoulder joints/blades during maximum elevation with stabilization of the serratus anterior. If the elevation capabilities are limited, there is a strengthening of the deltoid muscle.

Execution: 50x
The arms alternately perform a small up- / downward swimming stroke.

Common Mistakes:
The upper body loses its stability and starts swinging along.
The shoulders are pulled up toward the ears.
The elbows move further apart.
The movement is performed mostly at the end of the individual range of motion, making it discontinuous and less precise.

Modifications or Variations:
Place the legs in front of the Box or next to the Cadillac on Reformer Boxes.

Contraindications/Risks: -

18. Butterfly Straight Back (T)
1/2

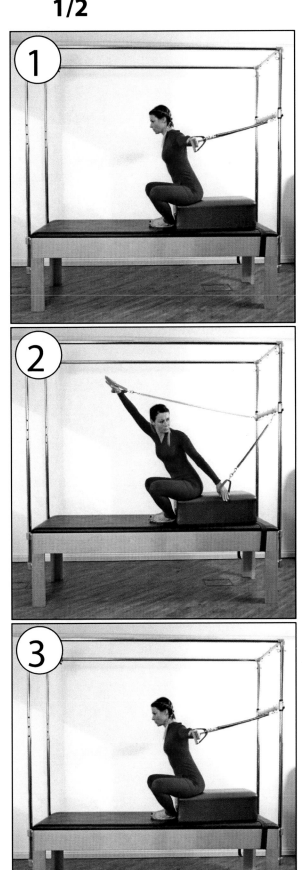

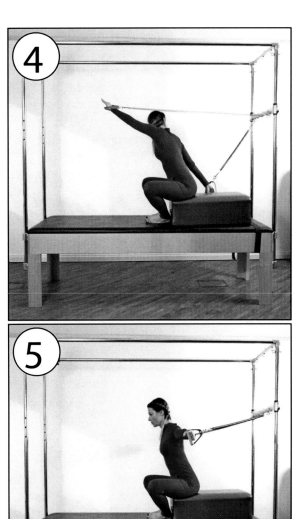

18. Butterfly Straight Back (T)
2/2

Setup:
Sitting, with a straight back and leaned forward. Both arms are opened to the sides.

Purpose of the Exercise:
Mobilization of the entire spine while rotating with low resistance.
Strengthening of the oblique abdominal muscles and the deltoid.
Coordinative training of the shoulder stabilizers.
Stretching of the side of the torso that one turns away from.

Execution: 3 sets
Beginning at the bottom, the upper body rotates to the right while the pelvis remains stable. Meanwhile, the right arm is lowered and rotated inward. The right palm faces the Box. Simultaneously, the left arm is raised up on the side and the palm faces in the direction of the rotation. The chest and head perform the rotation as far as possible. Look to the back.

Common Mistakes:
The shoulder of the upward stretched arm is pulled up.

Modifications or Variations:
Place the legs in front of the Box or next to the Cadillac on Reformer Boxes.

Contraindications/Risks: -

19. Spine Twist (T)

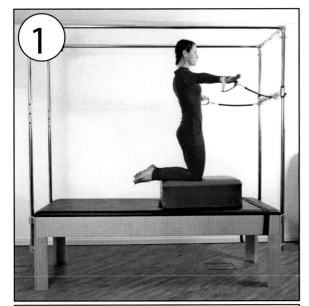

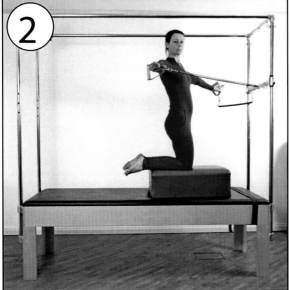

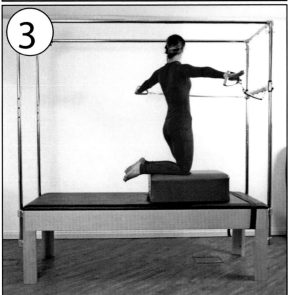

Setup:
Kneeling, looking toward the spring attachments. The arms are stretched to the sides. The hands are either as in the close-up below or, traditionally, holding the handles with the thumbs.

Purpose of the Exercise:
Strengthening of the posterior deltoid and torso rotators.
Stabilization of the triceps.
Coordinative training of the core muscles.

Execution: 5 sets
The movement is similar to the Spine Twist on the mat. Start the rotation of the spine in the hips. Yet, the hips first turn differently than for the same exercise on the mat. Hold the arms steady in one line and turn them to one side, against the resistance of the spring. Rotate the head slightly further than the chest.

Common Mistakes:
The hips move from side to side.
Excessive movement of the arms that exceeds the upper body rotation.

Modifications or Variations:
The exercise becomes easier, the more centrally one kneels on the Box.
The thumbs hold the handles.

Contraindications/Risks: -

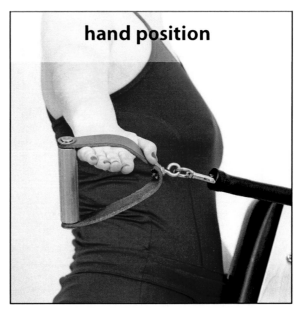

hand position

20. Swakatee (T)
Alternatively: Swaquity/Swockety/Swakkiti

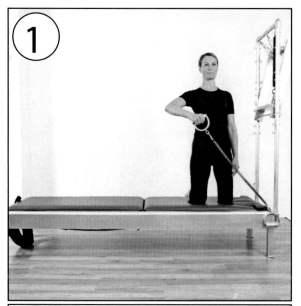

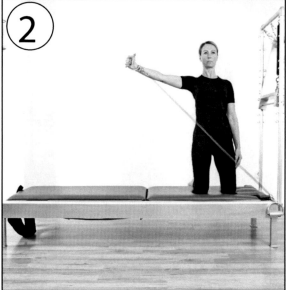

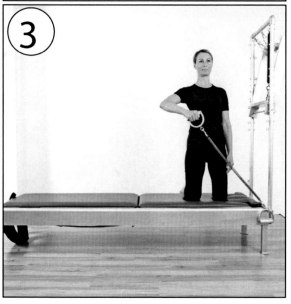

Setup:
Kneeling sideways on the Cadillac mat. The outer arm is at shoulder height and bent so that the hand is in front of the chest or of the opposite shoulder.

Purpose of the Exercise:
Strengthening of the posterior deltoid muscle and triceps.
Stabilization of the torso.

Execution: 4x per side
The outer arm is moved outward in a flowing motion as though opening a large door. Similar to a back fist strike. The arm is then moved back in the same manner.
Switch sides after the fourth repetition.

Common Mistakes:
The movement of the arm is divided into two single movements: elbow strike and then extension of the arm. This way, more strain is put on the elbow joint.

Modifications or Variations:
The head turns in the direction of the hand during the fourth repetition.

Contraindications/Risks: -

21. Shaving up the side of the head (T)

Alternatively: Shaving Side Arm / Uppa

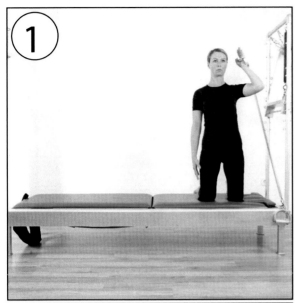

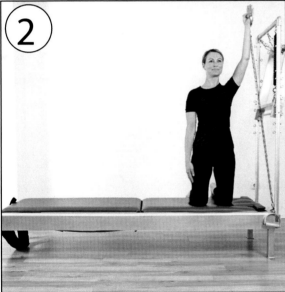

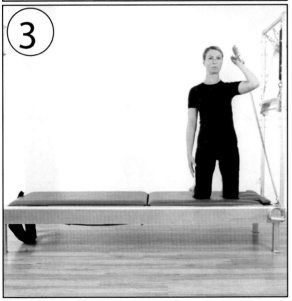

Setup:

Kneeling sideways on the Cadillac mat.
Place the hand of the arm that is closer to the spring attachments at ear height with the elbow facing outward.

Purpose of the Exercise:

Strengthening of the entire deltoid muscle and triceps with regard to constant control of the torso.

Execution: 4x per side

Stretch the inner arm up in a straight line from the outside of the shoulder until the maximum extension is reached. Then lower it back to the ear.
Switch sides after the fourth repetition.

Common Mistakes:

The arm deviates from the "ideal" line toward the side or the front. The shoulder loses its stability and moves toward the ear.

Modifications or Variations: -

Contraindications/Risks: -

22. Swakatee & Shaving Side Arm (T)

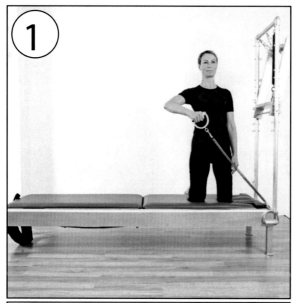

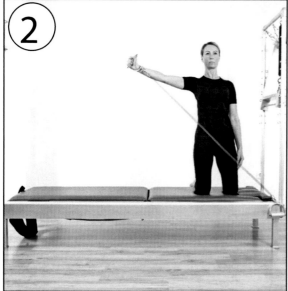

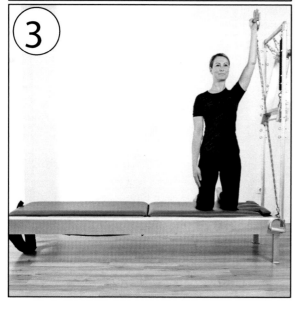

Setup:
Kneeling sideways on the Cadillac mat. The arm that is further away from the spring attachments is at shoulder level and bent so that the hand is in front of the chest or opposite shoulder.

Purpose of the Exercise:
Strengthening of the deltoid muscle and triceps with regard to constant control of the torso.

Execution: 3x per side
Cross Arm Pull: The outer arm is moved to the side in a flowing motion as though opening a large door. The head follows the motion and turns so that it faces the extended arm. The arm is moved back in the same manner.

Then switch hands and arms.

Shaving: Stretch the inner arm up in a straight line from the outside of the shoulder until its maximum extension is reached, then lower it back to the ear.

Switch hands and arms again.
Switch sides after the third repetition of the set.

Common Mistakes:
Cross Arm Pull: The movement of the arm is divided into two single movements - an elbow strike and then the extension of the arm. This way, more strain is put on the elbow joint.
Shaving: The arm deviates from the "ideal" line to the side or the front. The shoulder loses its stability and moves toward the ear.

Modifications or Variations: -

Contraindications/Risks: -

23. Profile (T)
Alternatively: Triceps

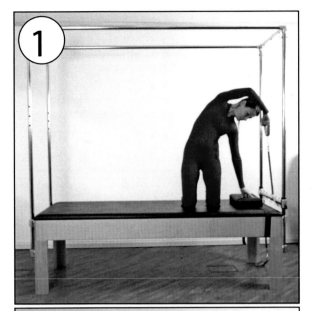

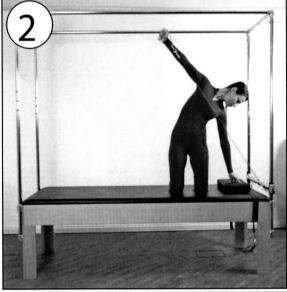

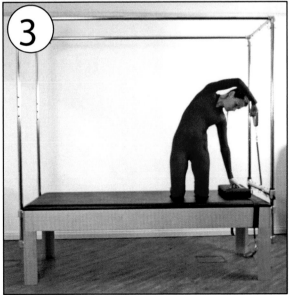

Setup:
Kneeling sideways on the Cadillac mat. The upper body is bent to the side with the spring attachments and the hand is placed on a Moon Box or Yoga block. Raise the outer arm and let it hang over the head, the hand points down and holds the handle of the anterior spring. The elbow is slightly bent. When performing the exercise, the hand should move only as close to the body as there is sufficient distance between the spring and the face.

Purpose of the Exercise:
Strengthening of the complete arm and shoulder muscles with a focus on the triceps.
Light stretching of the latissimus and oblique abdominal muscles.
Light mobilization of the lumbar/thoracic spine in the lateral flexion.

Execution: 4x per side
While remaining in the same position and without changing the height of the elbow, stretch the outer arm up to the side. Thereby the hand automatically turns so that it faces away from the body. Then bend the arm again to return it to the starting position.
Switch sides after the fourth repetition.

Common Mistakes:
The elbow of the outer arm moves up and down. This way, the triceps is less engaged.

Modifications or Variations: -

Contraindications/Risks: -

24. Lotus (T)

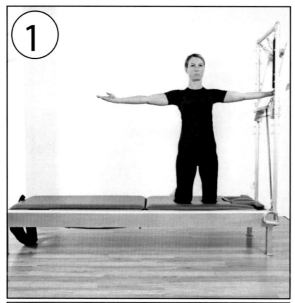

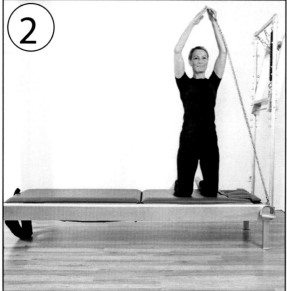

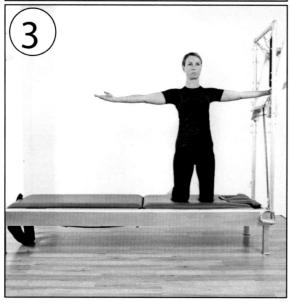

Setup:
Both hands are extended to the sides and the open palms face up. The hand that is closest to the spring attachments holds the handle of the anterior spring. The spring is put under minimal tension and does not hang loosely.

Purpose of the Exercise:
Strengthening of the deltoid.
Stabilization of the torso.

Execution: 4x per side
Move both arms upward and toward each other above the head with soft elbows. The fingertips of both hands touch. Both arms open to the sides until the starting position is reached again.
Switch sides after the fourth repetition.

Common Mistakes:
Trying to support the arm, the upper body moves away from the attachment of the spring.
The moving arm bends more strongly than the relaxed arm in order to facilitate the angle of strength.

Modifications or Variations: -

Contraindications/Risks: -

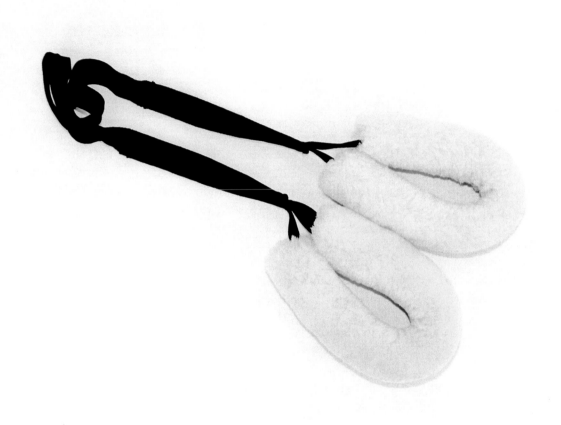

Fuzzies
Trapeze Bar
Trapeze Strap
Cadillac Frame

Preliminary Remarks for the Cadillac-Frame Exercises

There is a so-called "Traditional Ending" on the Cadillac, which typically consists of five exercises.

1. Breathing - which was introduced as exercise "29. Breathing (T)" in the Cadillac Manual part 1

2. Spread Eagle

3. Pull Ups

4. Hanging Pull Ups

5. Half Hanging/Full Hanging

Exercise 2 to 5 are presented in this part of the manual.

In addition to the exercises on the Cadillac frame that are listed above, there are other very demanding stretches, rotations in full hanging and exercises such as "The Squirrel". What they all have in common is that you should never do these exercises without an experienced Pilates instructor next to you and that they are not suitable for every Pilates practitioner. Hence, they are intentionally not presented here.

The traditional Cadillac exercises were complemented by, for example, the short Box series of the Reformer, which can also be performed well on the Cadillac or Tower with only a few compromises and is a useful addition, particularly for Tower group classes.

1. Kneeling Ballet Stretches (T)
1/3

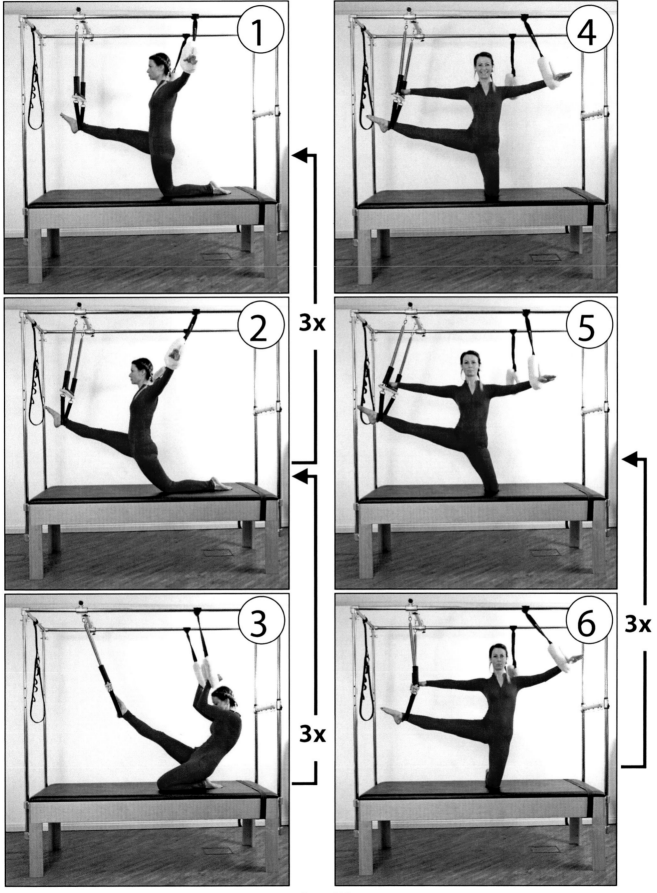

1. Kneeling Ballet Stretches (T)
2/3

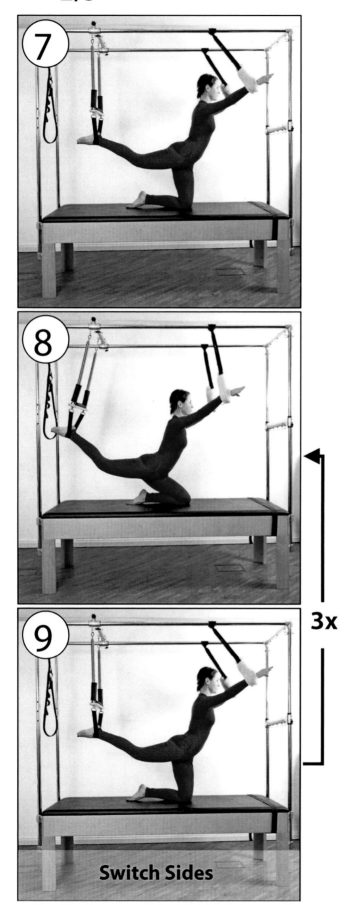

7

8

3x

9

Switch Sides

1. Kneeling Ballet Stretches (T) 3/3

Setup:

Adjust the distance between the Fuzzies and the Trapeze in such a way that the ankle of the right stretched leg in the Fuzzies can be placed on the Trapeze Strap at a 90 degree angle, while kneeling with the arms stretched out in a T-position. If possible, adjust the length of the Trapeze Strap so that the exercise can be performed in a relaxed manner. The less stretched, the deeper. Alternatively, hang the Trapeze lower with additional carabiners.
Stretch the hands through the Fuzzies so that the wrists rest in the Fuzzies.

Purpose of the Exercise:

Stretch of the hip flexors, leg backsides and inner thighs.

Execution: each position 3-5x as described

Image 1 -3: At the beginning of the exercise, push forward with the hip and back again. Repeat 3x - 5x.
Image 2 - 3: After pushing the hip forward, return to the starting position and bring the elbows in front of the body, the palms facing the head. Form fists and flex the wrists. Now sit down on the rear, left leg and round the back. Come back up, spread out the arms and push forward from your hips. Repeat 3x - 5x.
Image 4: From the starting position, turn the left leg and then the whole body by 90 degrees. While the left hand remains in the Fuzzie, the right hand moves to the Trapeze Bar.
Image 5 - 6: First push the hip to the right. At the same time, the left leg is automatically abducted on the Cadillac. Then push it to the left, moving outward, slightly beyond the starting position so that a light lateral flexion to the right occurs.
Image 7: Once again, first turn the left leg and then the whole body by 90 degrees. The left hand switches to the next fuzzy and the hand from the Trapeze Bar switches to the now empty fuzzy.
Image 8 - 9: Push the hip backward first and then come forward as far as possible.

Common Mistakes:

The starting position is too challenging. Subsequently, the pelvis is always tilted to one side.
Too much effort is used for support and holding, out of fear of falling over.

Modifications or Variations:

Instead of being able to touch the Fuzzies during the exercise in pictures 4, 5, 6, the upper horizontal Cadillac bar can also be grabbed whole or with just one hand.
Instead of being able to hold the Fuzzies during the exercise in pictures 7, 8, 9, the two front vertical Cadillac poles can also be grabbed in case of less flexibility.
Perform the exercise while standing, then with the leg on the Trapeze Bar.

Contraindications/Risks: -

2. Standing Ballet Stretches (T)
1/3

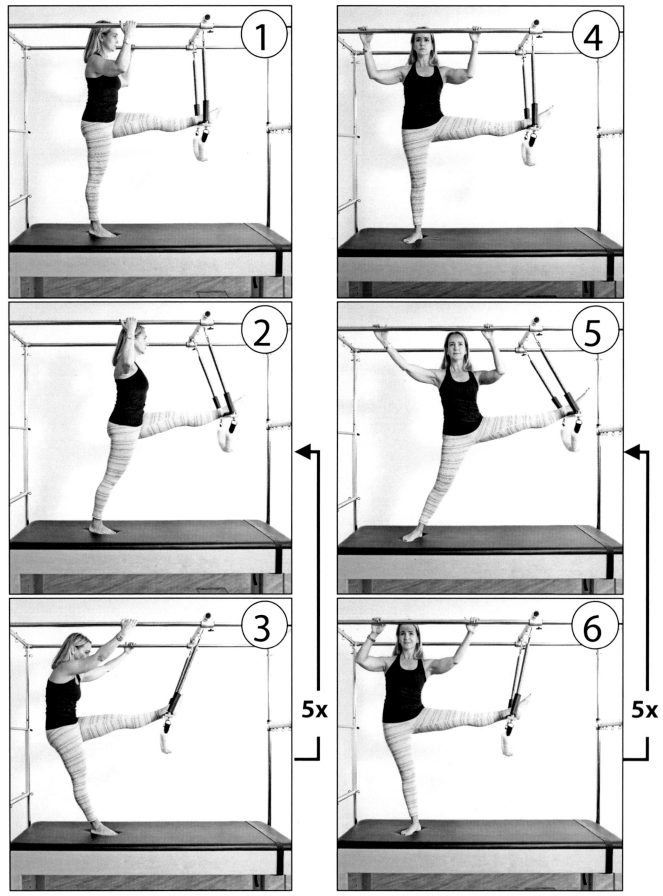

5x

5x

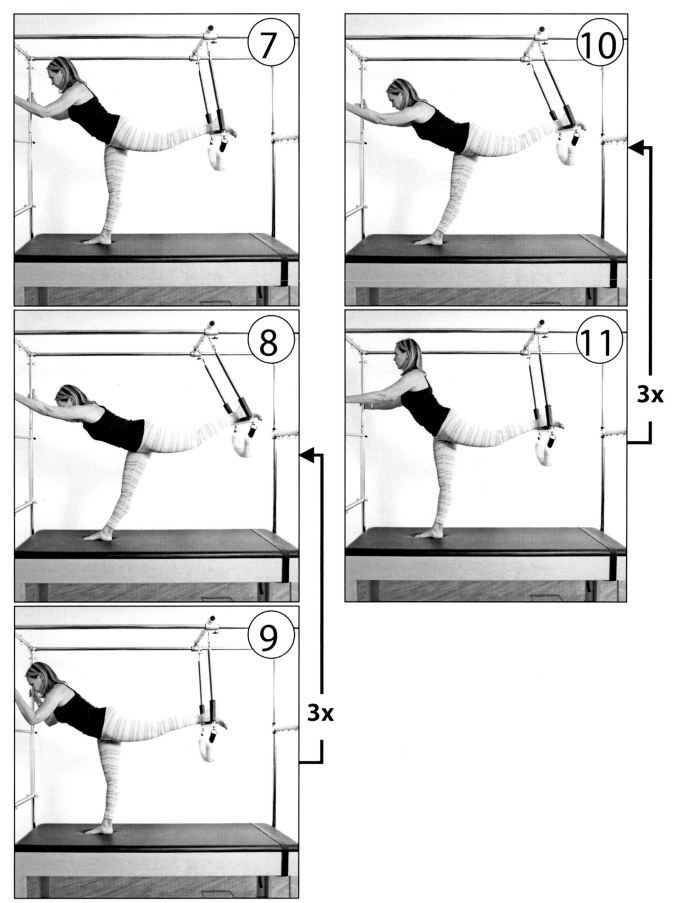

2. Standing Ballet Stretches (T)
3/3

Setup:
Standing on the Cadillac, looking at the Trapeze. The left leg is on the Trapeze. The hands hold the upper frame of the Cadillac from the outside with outstretched arms. The left stretched leg lies in the center of the Trapeze at the Achilles tendon. Select the distance to the Trapeze so that a 90 degree angle to the standing leg is reached. Stand upright.

Purpose of the Exercise:
Stretch of the hip flexors, leg backsides and inner thighs.

Execution: repeat each position 3x -5x
Image 1 -3: Push the entire body forward. Keep the upper body upright. Then bring the body back a little further than it was in the starting position. Repeat 3x - 5x.

Image 4: Keep the leg on the Trapeze and turn to the right. The hands rest on the Trapeze attachment and the crossbar of the Cadillac frame. Stretch both legs out as far as possible.

Image 5 - 6: First push the hip to the left and swing the Trapeze along accordingly. Then push the hip to the right and move it outward slightly beyond the starting position so that a light lateral flexion occurs. Repeat 3x - 5x.

Image 7: Again leave the left leg on the Trapeze Bar and turn the whole body by 90 degrees, now looking away from the Trapeze. Hold the vertical bars of the Cadillac with the hands. The ankle lies on the Trapeze. Stretch both legs out as far as possible.

Image 8 - 9: Begin by pushing the hips back and then come back with the body. Do not come into the extension yet. Repeat 3x.

Image 10 - 11: Push the hip back again and then come back while in the extension with stretched arms. Repeat 3x.

Common Mistakes:
The starting position is too challenging. Hence, the pelvis is always slightly tilted to one side.

Modifications or Variations:
For very small people the Trapeze Strap can also be used for the foot and the Fuzzies Straps to grip.

Contraindications/Risks:
Danger of luxation in case of fresh hip endoprostheses.

3. Spread Eagle (T)
1/2

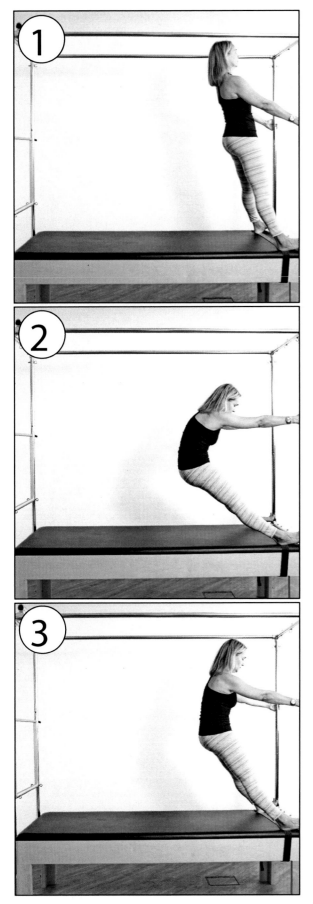

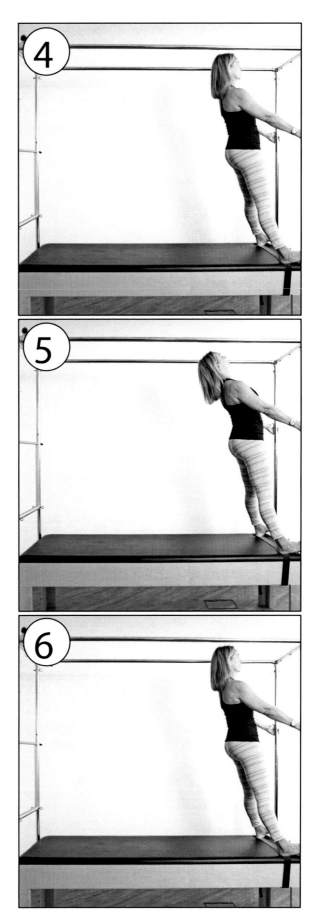

3. Spread Eagle (T)
2/2

Setup:
Standing, looking toward the open end of the Cadillac. The feet are placed against the vertical poles or the Kuna Board/Spread Eagle Board at their balls. The tips of the toes end at the top edge when using the Kuna Board. The heels are on the Cadillac mat. The legs are in outward rotation.

The body leans backward in a slight stretch. With stretched arms, the hands hold the vertical bars. The height of the grip naturally results where the hands grip with relaxed shoulders, downward stretched arms and the body leaning backward. Each change in height alters slightly how far the body can go into the extension. The pelvic height essentially determines the extension of the thoracic spine. From the navel to the shoulder there is more full body extension.

Purpose of the Exercise:
Mobilization of the spine.
Stretch of the backside of the body.

Execution: 3x - 5x
Pull the abdomen inward and bring the head and pubic bone together to form a large arch. The movement is directed by the navel. The arms and legs remain stretched. The body part that is brought furthest back is the lower back, not the buttocks.

Pull the scapulae downward to straighten the body diagonally again. From the complete stretch of the body, following the apex of the head, move the cervical and upper thoracic spine into an overstretch.

Return to upright position.

Repeat 3x - 5x.

Common Mistakes:
The buttocks direct the backward movement.

The extension is performed without internal abdominal tension and individual vertebral elements are overstrained.

The movement is performed unnaturally.

Modifications or Variations:
Instead of the traditional version, perform exercise "4. Spread Eagle Variation (M)".

Perform the exercise on a Kuna Board instead of at the poles. The tiptoes end at the upper edge.

During the exercise the feet change their position: At the beginning the feet are placed against the poles or a Kuna Board. On the way back, rotate the legs and feet outward so that the feet pass the vertical poles or the Kuna Board in a large "V".

Perform the whole exercise with the legs in an outward rotation.

Contraindications/Risks: -

4. Spread Eagle Variation (M)
1/2

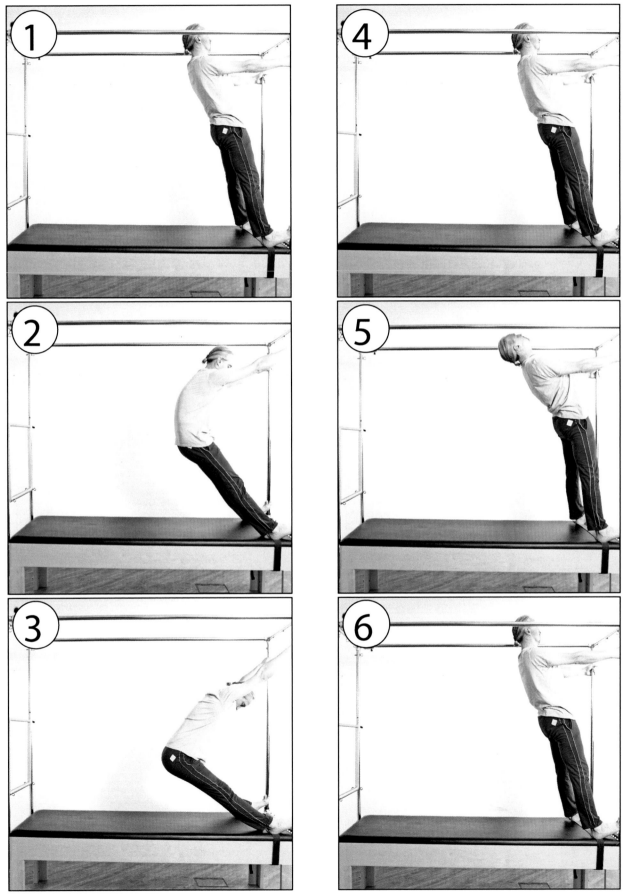

4. Spread Eagle Variation (M)
2/2

Setup:
Standing, looking toward the open end of the Cadillac. The feet are placed against the vertical poles or the Kuna Board/Spread Eagle Board at their balls. The tips of the toes end at the top edge when using the Kuna Board. The heels are on the Cadillac mat. The legs are in outward rotation.
Each change in height alters slightly how far the body can go into the extension. The pelvic height essentially determines the extension of the thoracic spine. From the navel to the shoulder there is more full body extension.

Purpose of the Exercise:
Mobilization of the spine.
Stretch of the front and back of the body.

Execution: 3x - 5x
Pull the abdomen inward and bring the head and pubic bone closer toward each other to form a large arch. The movement is directed by the navel. The arms and legs remain stretched. At the lowest possible position, tilt the pelvis anteriorly and stretch the upper part of the body to form a long-seat position.
Pull the scapulae downward to straighten the body up diagonally again. From the complete extension of the body, following the vertex of the head, push the pelvis forward and overstretch the entire spine.
Maintain the inner abdominal tension.
Repeat 3x - 5x.

Common Mistakes:
The extension is performed without inner abdominal tension and individual vertebral elements are overstrained.

Modifications or Variations:
Perform the exercise on a Kuna Board instead of at the poles. The tiptoes end at the upper edge.
During the exercise the feet change their position: At the beginning the feet are placed against the poles or a Kuna Board. On the way back, rotate the legs and feet outward so that the feet pass the vertical poles or the Kuna Board in a large "V".
Perform the whole exercise with the legs in an outward rotation.

Contraindications/Risks: -

5. Reverse Spread Eagle (M)
1/2

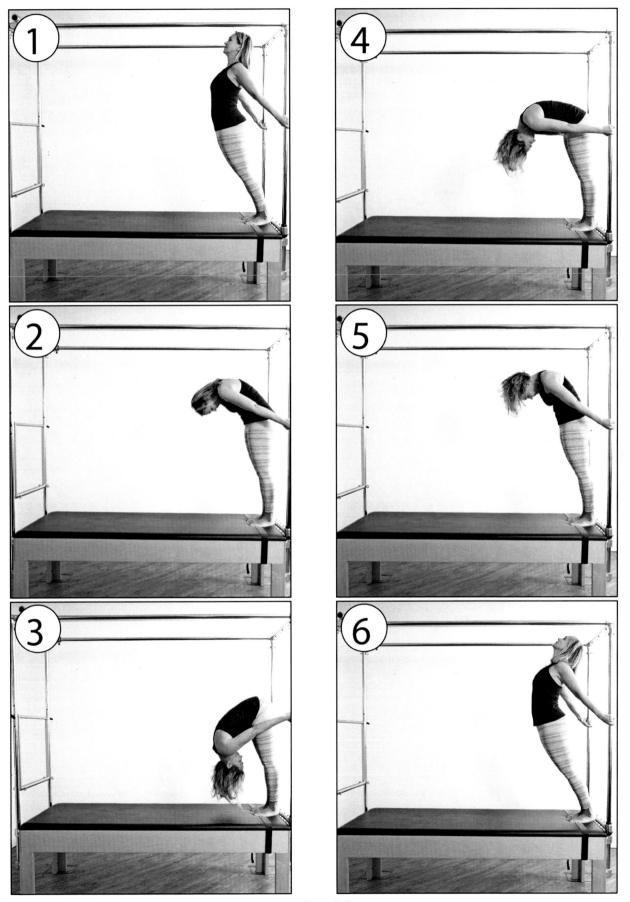

5. Reverse Spread Eagle (M)
2/2

Setup:
Standing, looking into the Cadillac and away from the open end. The feet are placed on the Kuna Board/Spread Eagle Board in a small "V" to reduce the risk of slipping. The hands reach backward to the vertical poles. The position of the hands may change during the exercise. With stretched arms and legs push the pelvis forward out of the standing position, the chest and head pointing toward the ceiling. Maintain internal abdominal tension.

Purpose of the Exercise:
Mobilization of the spine.
Stretch of the front and back of the body.

Execution: 3x - 5x

Following the vertex of the head, roll down vertebra by vertebra.
At the lowest point let the body hang forward into the arms.
Beginning with a posterior pelvic tilt, roll back up and straighten the body vertebra by vertebra into the star position.
Pay attention to any feeling of dizziness and wait until it is over before the next repetition.

Repeat 3x - 5x.

Common Mistakes:
The extension is performed without internal abdominal tension and individual vertebral elements are overstrained.

Modifications or Variations: -

Contraindications/Risks: -

6. Hanging Pull Ups (T)
1/2

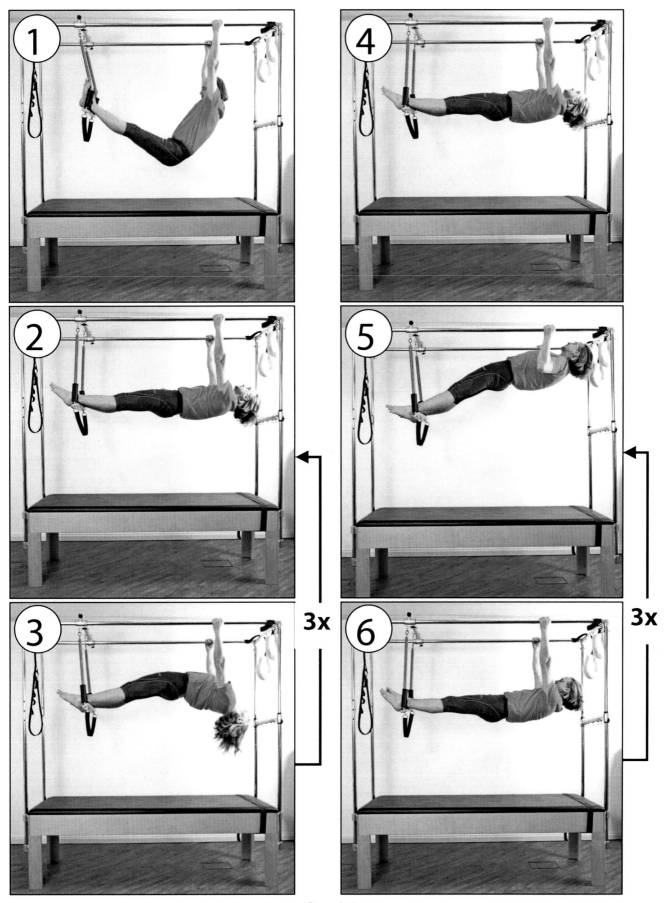

3x

3x

6. Hanging Pull Ups (T)
2/2

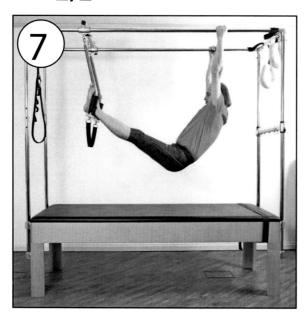

Setup:
The hands grip the roof of the Cadillac from the outside, with the fingers on the outside and the thumbs inside (human grip). Ankles on the Trapeze Bar, feet around the springs of the Trapeze Bar. Hang loosely in this position for a few seconds. The distance between the handle and the Trapeze Bar can be adjusted according to individual experience. The Trapeze Bar should hang as vertically as possible when the body is stretched.

Purpose of the Exercise:
Hanging Image 1 and 7: Traction of various joints with the focus on the shoulders and elbows. Stretch of the backside of the body.
Plank Image 2: Full body tension and strengthening of the hands and forearm muscles.
Extension Image 3: Strengthening of the back extensors and stretching of the front.
Pull-Up Image 4-5: Strengthening of the brachialis, biceps, brachii and brachioradialis.

Execution:
Stretch the feet and the body. From there, come into an overextension which is evenly spread across the spine. Return into the stretched position. The Trapeze is not moved throughout the exercise.
Repeat 3x.
Pull yourself up as far as possible from the stretched position and come back down. The Trapeze is still not moved.
Repeat 3x.
Finally, hang loosely for a few seconds again.

Common Mistakes:
The Trapeze is moved during the pull-up.

Modifications or Variations: -

Contraindications/Risks: -

7.   Pull Ups (T)

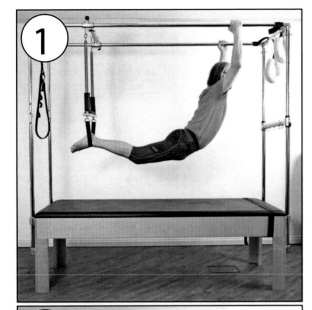

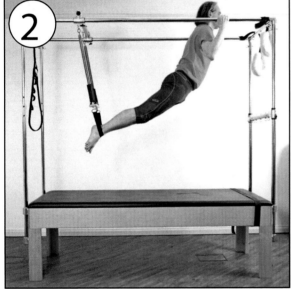

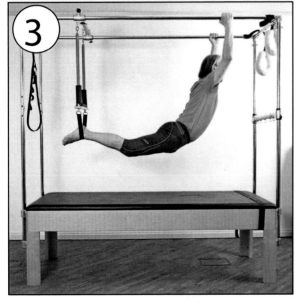

Setup:

Standing with the back toward the Trapeze. The hands grip the roof of the Cadillac from the outside. Place the ankles on the Trapeze Strap one after the other. Stretch out the arms and the body as a whole is in a well spread overextension supported by the abdominal muscles. The distance between the handle and the Trapeze Bar can be adjusted according to individual experience. The Trapeze Bar should hang as vertically as possible when the body is stretched.

Purpose of the Exercise:

Strengthening of the pectoralis (major and minor), latissimus dorsi, lower part of the trapezius, brachialis, biceps brachii and brachioradialis.
Strengthening of the hands and forearm muscles.
Stretch of the entire front of the body.

Execution: 3x - 5x

Pull the body up as far as possible by bending the arms, then come back down. The Trapeze is not moved throughout the exercise.
Repeat 3x -5x.

Common Mistakes:

The Trapeze is moved during the pull-up.
Hanging with a hollow back.
The head sinks in between the shoulders.

Modifications or Variations:

To learn the exercise, place one bent leg on the Cadillac and lay the other leg onto the Trapeze Strap. Lunge. Stretch and bend the standing leg several times. The arms bend and stretch as well. Do not move the Trapeze. Depending on the focus of the exercise, either use the force from the arms to pull up or use the leg muscles. Then switch legs.
As an alternative preliminary exercise, place one leg in the Trapeze Strap, then both legs, then immediately pull out one leg again and bring it forward.

Contraindications/Risks:

In case of problems in the back or in the shoulder, omit the exercise.

8. Half Hanging & Full Hanging (T)
1/3

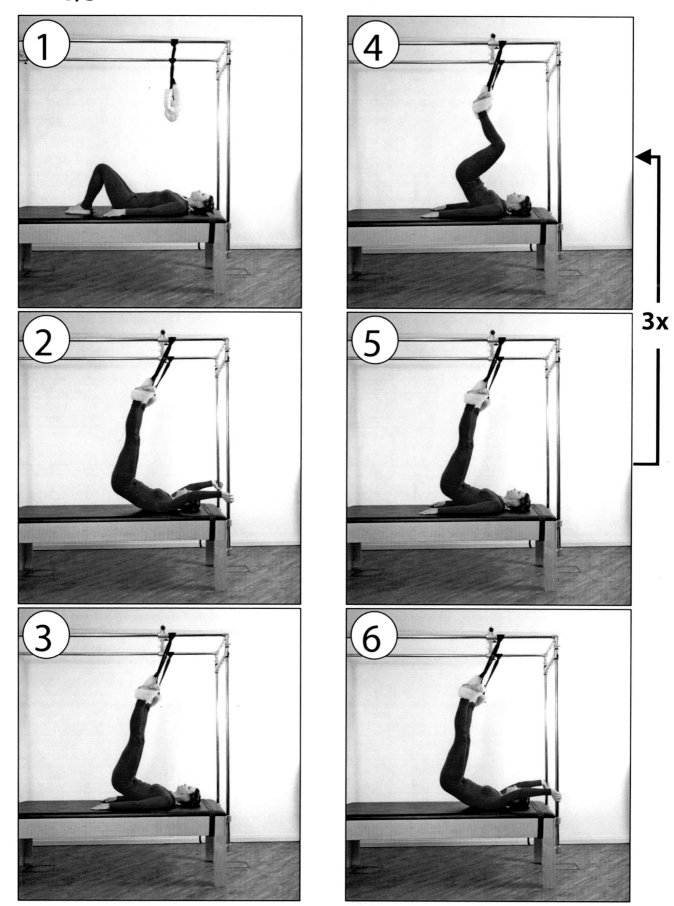

3x

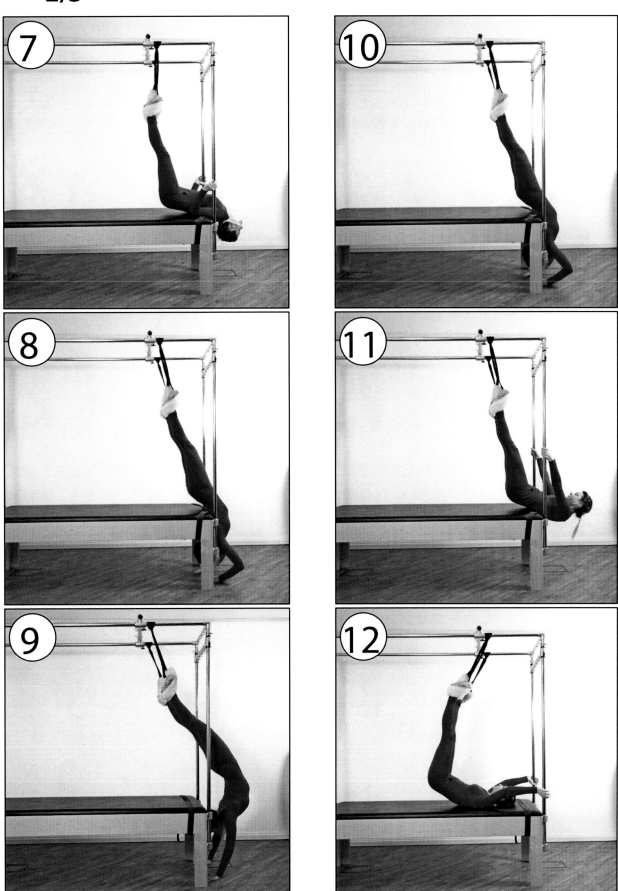

8. Half Hanging & Full Hanging (T)
3/3

Setup:

Position the Fuzzies one ell away from the lateral bars of the Cadillac. The Trapeze attachment can be used to ensure that the two Fuzzies are hanging at the same height. Lie with the head at the end of the Cadillac. Roll up and slip into the Fuzzies with the feet. Tighten the Fuzzies by rotating the legs. The Legs are slightly rotated outward. Flex the feet to make sure not to slip out of the Fuzzies. Grip the vertical Cadillac poles with the hands slightly above shoulder height and push away until a distance of one arm-length is reached.

Purpose of the Exercise:

Traction of various joints.
Stretch of the front and back of the body.

Execution:

As a preliminary exercise - Half Hanging: Bend the knees, slightly opened to the sides, and then stretch the legs again. This raises the spine and lowers it as much as possible while straightening the legs. Repeat 3x - 5x. Grip the vertical Cadillac poles with the hands slightly above shoulder height and pull the body across the Cadillac edge until it hangs down completely. On modern Cadillacs without a bar at ankle level, place the hands on the ground for support, if possible. Come into an overstretched handstand. Alternatively, use a Kuna Board or two yoga blocks to reach a higher position with the hands. On classic Cadillacs with a ledge, place the hands on the ledge and enter the overstretched handstand.
Bend the arms again, grip the vertical bars with the hands, lift the head and come up. Pull the body back onto the Cadillac and come out of the loops. Caution, help may be needed to get out of the Fuzzies.

Common Mistakes: -

Modifications or Variations: -

Contraindications/Risks: -

9. Swan (M)

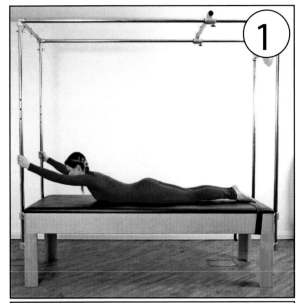

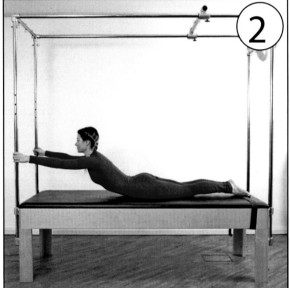

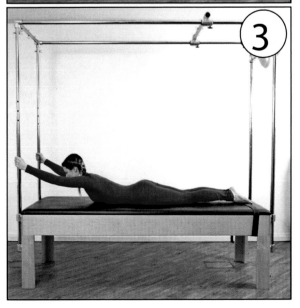

Setup:
Prone position, one arm-length away from the vertical bars of the Cadillac frame.
The hands hold the vertical Cadillac poles above shoulder height.
At the start of the exercise there is already a slight extension of the thoracic spine and the head is slightly lifted, looking down at the mat.

Purpose of the Exercise:
Strengthening of the back extensors.
Stretch of the latissimus dorsi, teres major and pectoralis major.
Mobilization of the shoulder joint/blade.

Execution: 3x - 7x
Pull in the abdomen to distribute the strain on the spine as evenly as possible. Actively pull the scapulae downward. Lift the head and chest and come up as high as possible. Then lower the head and chest back to the starting position.
Repeat 3x -7x.

Common Mistakes:
The shoulders are pulled up toward the ears.
The elbows are widened.
Too much strength is taken from the chest muscles.

Modifications or Variations: -

Contraindications/Risks:
Omit the exercise in case of shoulder problems.

10. Tower Prep (Alan Herdman)
1/2

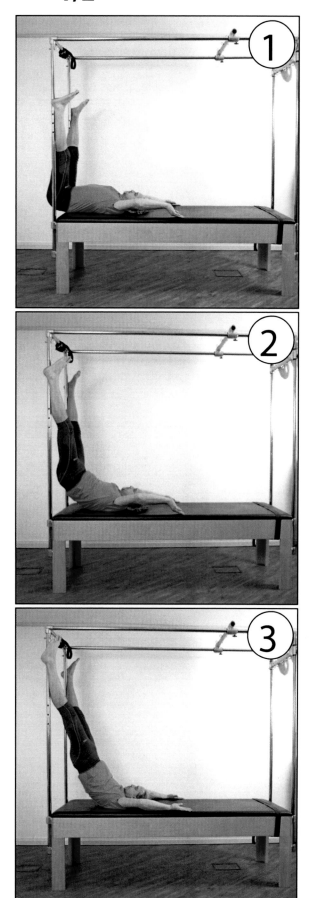

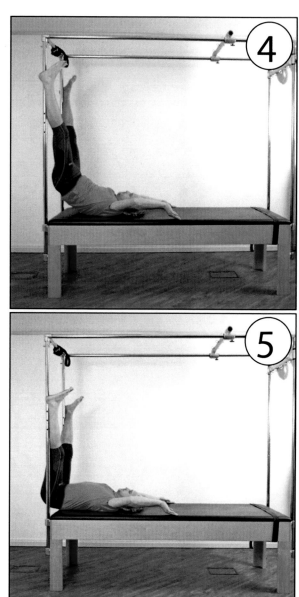

10. Tower Prep (Alan Herdman)
2/2

Setup:
Lying with the buttocks over the Cadillac edge of the open side, or the side with the fewest eyelets, which could interfere with the exercise. Open the legs with the calves on the vertical poles, place the inner sides of the heels against the outer sides of the poles. Stretch the arms past the head, out on the Cadillac mat. If this is not possible due to shoulder constraints, place the arms sideways next to the upper body and hips.

Purpose of the Exercise:
Mobilization of the spine as an alternative for more challenging exercises such as the Tower.
Strengthening of the lower abdominal muscles.

Execution: 3x - 5x
With stretched legs, roll up vertebra by vertebra. Use the vertical bars of the Cadillac for guidance, but do not push against them unnecessarily. Make sure that the head is not pressed into the Cadillac mat in the end position and that it could still be lifted.
Slowly roll down vertebra by vertebra with the legs stretched out.

Common Mistakes:
Pushing away from the vertical bars with the legs too strongly and thereby applying too much pressure to the shoulder and cervical spine.

Modifications or Variations:
If the sliding along the bars is uncomfortable with the lower legs left bare, alternatively place a cloth or sliding pad between the lower leg and the bar.

Contraindications/Risks: -

11. Full Circle (Guillotine) (T)
1/4

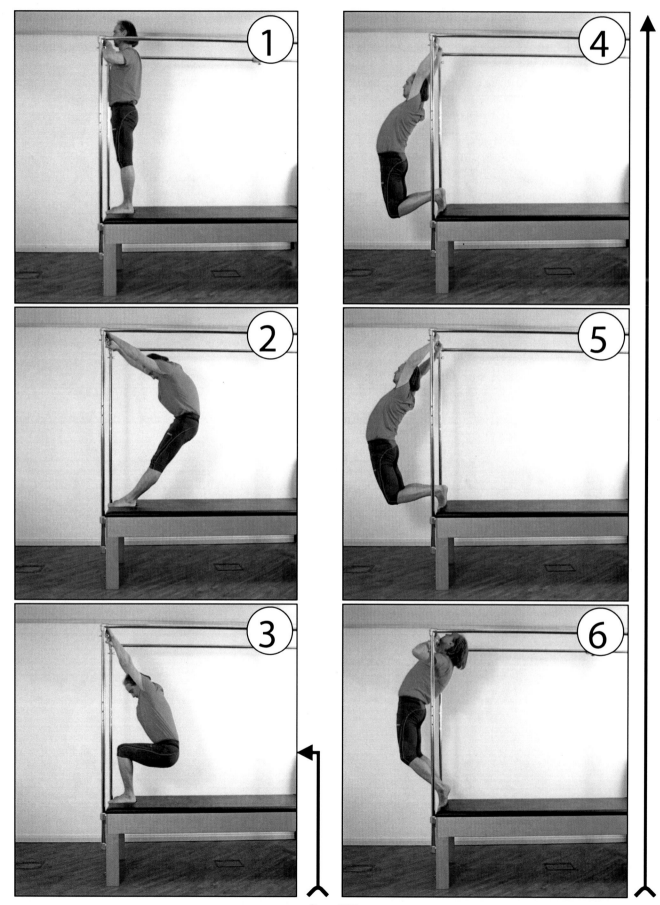

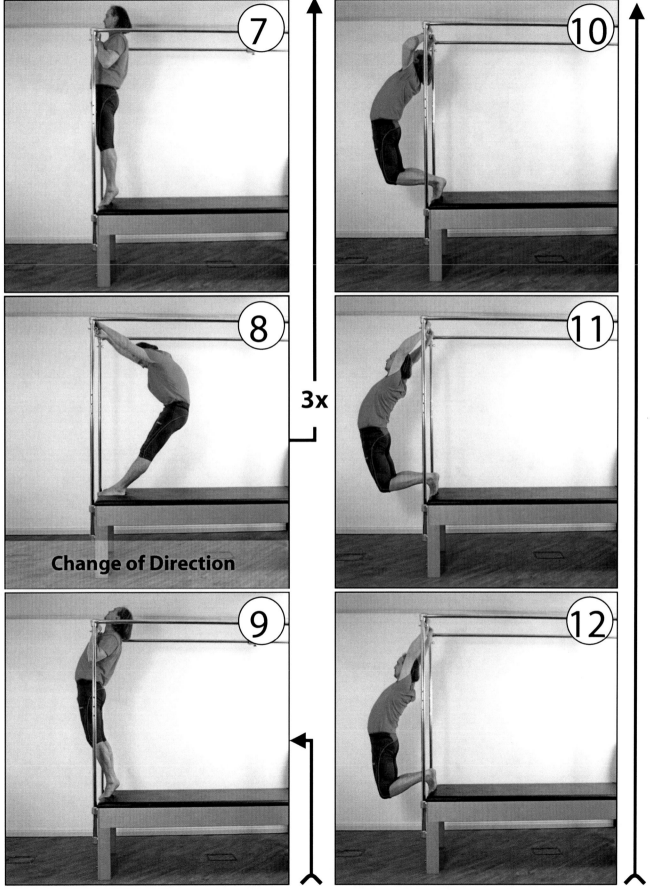

Change of Direction

3x

11. Full Circle (Guillotine) (T)
3/4

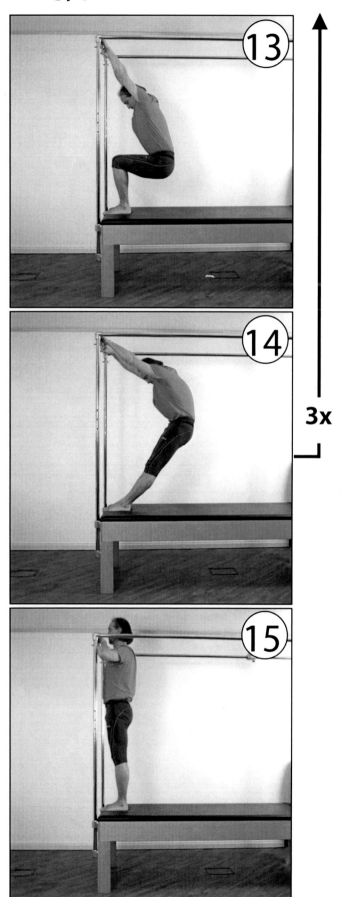

11. Full Circle (Guillotine) (T)
4/4

Setup:

The exercise originates from the Guillotine, where one stands on the movable bar and holds on to the fixed bar at the top. On the Guillotine, the distance is smaller, the upper bar is rather at chest height, and therefore the exercise is somewhat easier than with the greater distance on the Cadillac.

Stand at the open end of the Cadillac with the toes on and very slightly across the edge. Hold on to the crossbar of the Cadillac roof with the hands shoulder-wide apart.

Purpose of the Exercise:

Stretch of the front and back of the body.
Mobilization of the entire spine.

Execution: 3x per direction

Image 2: Round backward. Viewed from the side, there is a Teaser, rotated by 90°.
Image 3: Bend the knees and transfer the weight into the hands.
Image 4: Bring the knees forward and down and already hang slightly over the edge of the Cadillac.
Image 5: Push the hips all the way to the front to bring the body into an overextension, supported by the abdominal muscles.
Image 6: Bend the arms and pull up the body with the chin, neck and chest close to the horizontal roof bar of the Cadillac. Slide across the bar as closely as possible.
Image 7: In the end position, stand on the tips of your toes as though pulling further up the next moment.
Image 8: Round the body again and hang through loosely toward the back. Teaser position.
Repeat 3x.

Image 9: Pull the body up toward the horizontal roof bar, as though doing a pull up on the bar. The body is already overstretching. Round backward. Viewed from the side, there is a Teaser , rotated by 90°.
Image 10 -11: Slowly, lower forward, gliding past the horizontal bar as closely as possible. Push the hip all the way to the front to bring the body into an overextension supported by the abdominal muscles.
Image 12-14: Bend the knees, bring the body backward, round it again and hang through loosely. Teaser position.
Repeat 3x.

Common Mistakes:

Uncertainty about the sequence and therefore imprecise execution.

Modifications or Variations:

In case of nervousness, first only carry out the movement from image 2 to image 3 until enough trust in one's own arm strength has been gained.

Contraindications/Risks:

In case of painful shoulder problems, the fear of pain may interfere with the exercise. In this case it is better to omit the exercise.

12. Leg Lifts (Guillotine) (T)
1/2

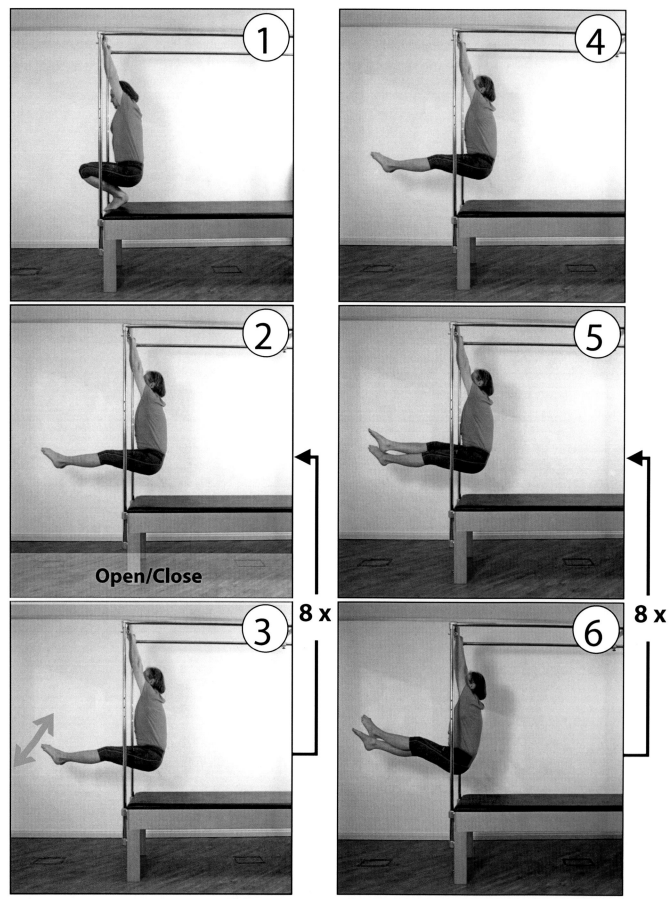

Open/Close

8 x

8 x

12. Leg Lifts (Guillotine) (T)
2/2

Setup:

The exercise originates from the work on the Guillotine.
Standing inside the Cadillac at the open end without a Push-Through-Bar. The hands grip the horizontal bar of the Cadillac roof shoulder-wide apart. Bend the legs until the upper body hangs from the arms. Then raise the legs until they are at a 90 degree angle to the torso and parallel to the floor.

Purpose of the Exercise:

Strengthening of the hand and forearm muscles, hip flexors, leg adductors and trunk muscles with the focus on the abdominal muscles.
Traction of the shoulders.

Execution:

Part 1: The legs perform small beats to the sides, opening and closing. Repeat up to 8 times.
Part 2: "Changements", instead of opening to the sides, the legs quickly alternate between up and down movements.

Common Mistakes:

Excessive rounding and giving up the torso stability.

Modifications or Variations:

Perform big leg circles instead of the beats.

Contraindications/Risks: -

13. Teaser 1 (T)
1/3

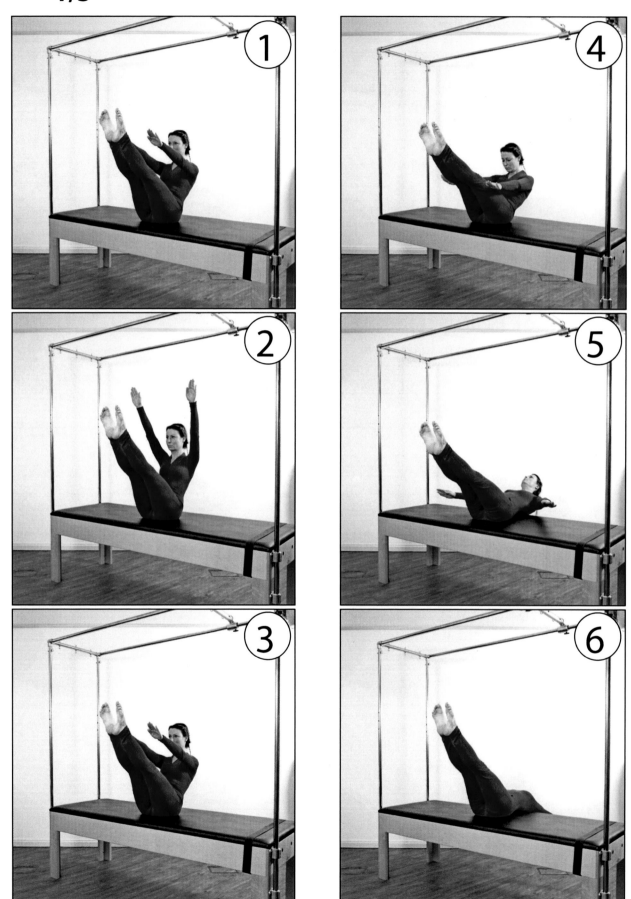

13. Teaser 1 (T)
2/3

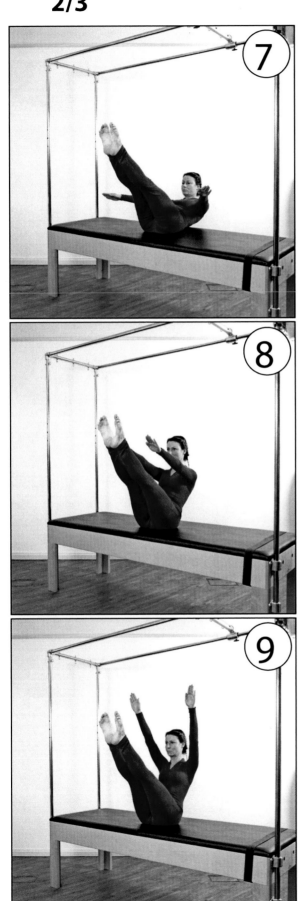

13. Teaser 1 (T)
3/3

Setup:
Sit diagonally on the Cadillac mat in the Teaser position. The height of the legs is individual. Use 45 degrees as a first approximation. The lumbar spine is rounded. Select the sitting position so that the tips of the shoulder blades are exactly above the edge of the Cadillac mat when rolled down backwards. Keep the arms parallel to the legs at the start, the palms face downward.

Purpose of the Exercise:
Strengthening of the hip flexors and the entire abdominal musculature.
Stretch of the abdominal and shoulder muscles and opening of the thoracic and cervical spine.

Execution: 3x - 7x
Stretch the arms up next to the head, the palms of the hands facing forward. Lower the arms and bring them down past the legs. Roll down slowly and in a controlled manner, keep the legs at 45 degrees. Open the arms and bring them to the back in a big circle. The thoracic spine and neck are in a controlled overextension. The arms are next to the head in the end position, if possible.
Come back the same way. The arms are opened to the sides again. Lift the head first and roll back up into the Teaser. Keep the legs at the same height at all times. Raise the arms again and place them next to the head. Start from Image 3 again to repeat the exercise.

Common Mistakes:
In the Teaser position, the lumbar spine is stretched, which is often a sign of a weak transversus abdominis. The legs do not hold any internal tension and the small "V" is given up.
The legs sink during exercise.

Modifications or Variations:
Instead of bringing the arms downward in a circular arc and then backward, the more demanding method is to keep the arms stretched up beside the head and then roll down directly.
At the end of the exercise Leg Circles: Lower the legs, open them at the bottom, pull them apart and then bring them up into the starting position in a "D". Repeat 3x - 5x, then change the direction.

Contraindications/Risks: -

14. Teaser 3 (T)
1/2

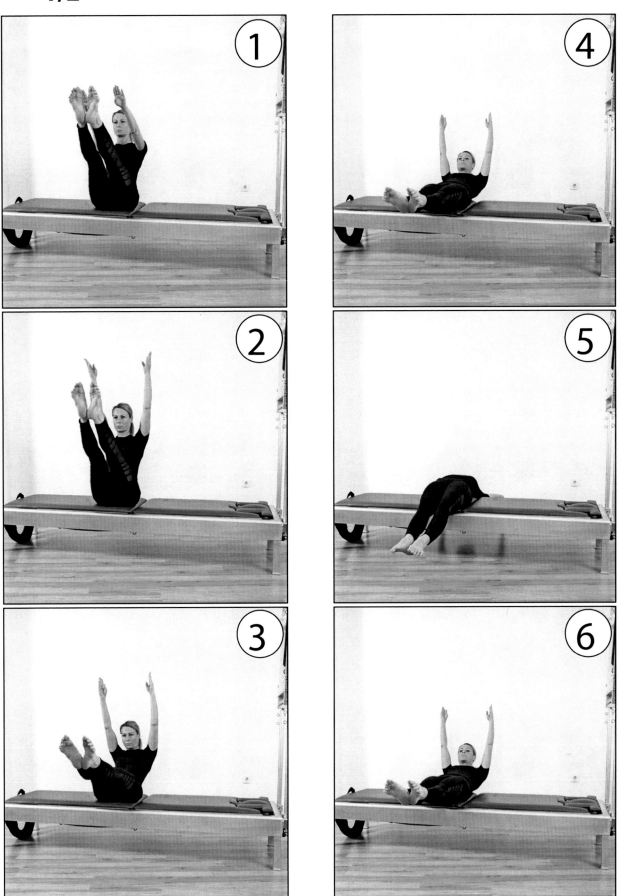

14. Teaser 3 (T)
2/2

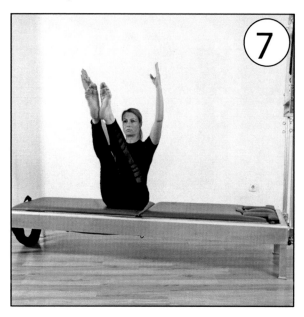

Setup:

Sit diagonally on the Cadillac mat in the Teaser position. Rounded lumbar spine. Choose a sitting position in which the tips of the shoulder blades are exactly above the edge of the Cadillac mat when rolled down. The arms are parallel to the legs at the start, the palms face downward.

Purpose of the Exercise:

Strengthening of the hip flexors and the entire abdominal musculature.
Stretch of the abdominal muscles, shoulder muscles and hip flexors.
Opening of the thoracic and cervical spine.

Execution: 3x - 7x

Raise the arms up next to the ears, the palms of the hands face forward. Roll down slowly and in a controlled manner with the arms next to the ears and simultaneously lower the legs. The head and feet remain at the same height. After reaching the horizontal, lower the legs and simultaneously roll down the thoracic spine and the head into a controlled overextension. The arms are next to the head in the end position, if possible. Maintain inner abdominal tension.

Come back the same way. Raise the arms first, then the head and roll back up into the Teaser. Raise the arms again and place them next to the head.

Common Mistakes:

In the Teaser position, the lumbar spine is stretched, which is often a sign of a weak transversus abdominis. The legs do not hold any internal tension and the small "V" is given up.

Modifications or Variations:

At the end of the exercise, perform leg circles: Lower the legs, open them at the bottom, pull them apart and then bring them up into the starting position in a "D". Repeat 3x - 5x, then change the direction.

Contraindications/Risks:

Danger of a hollow back while raising the legs.

15. Teaser & Log Roll (T)
   1/8

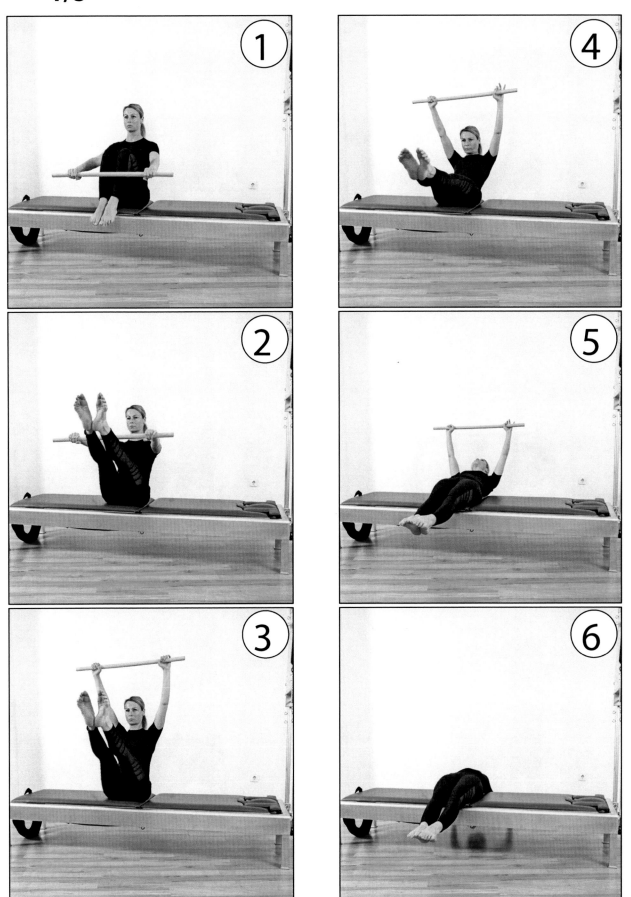

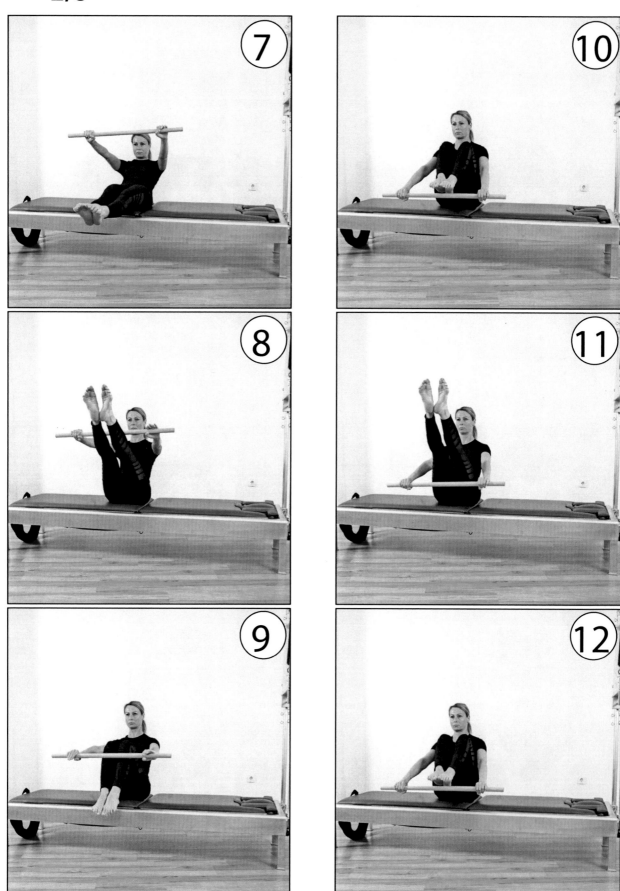

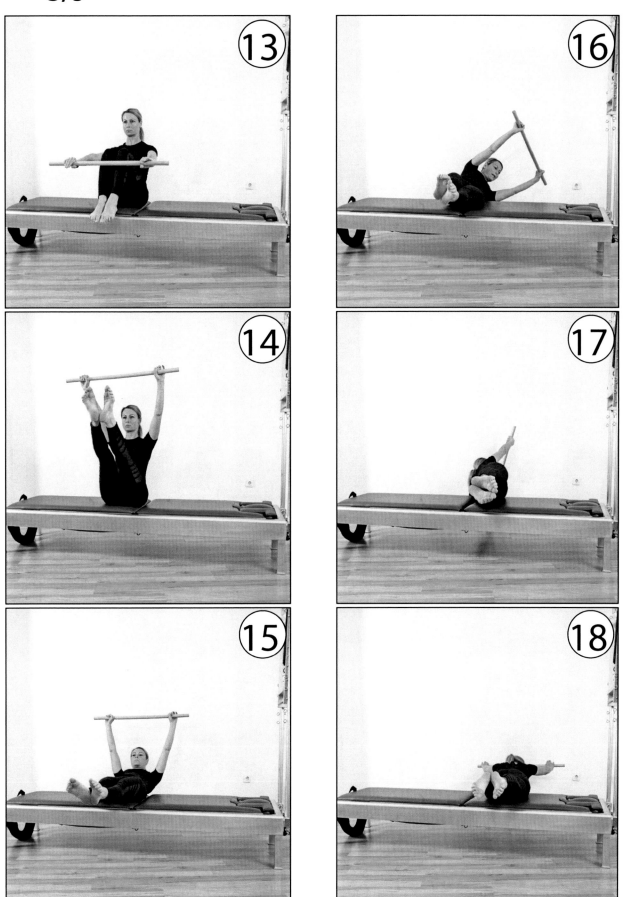

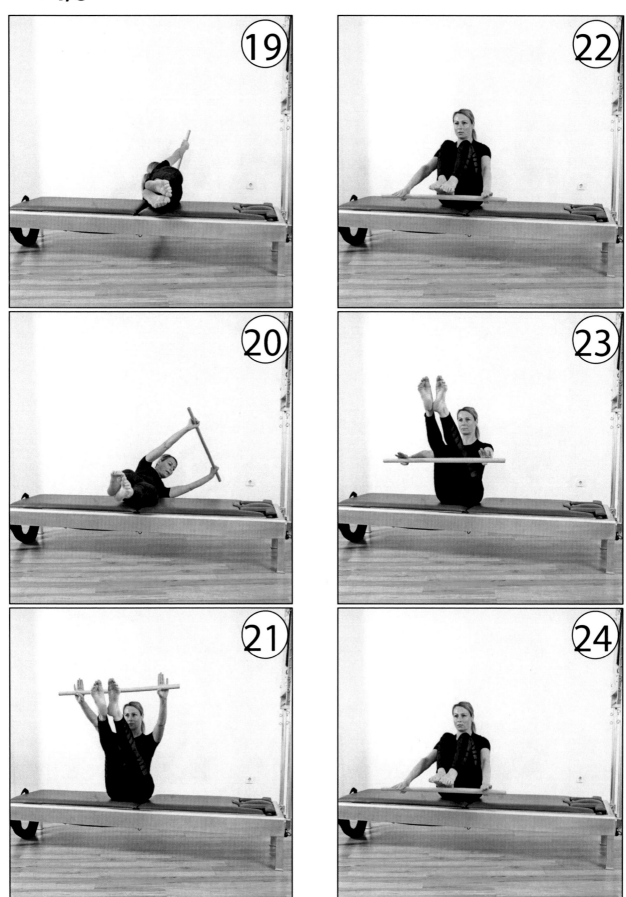

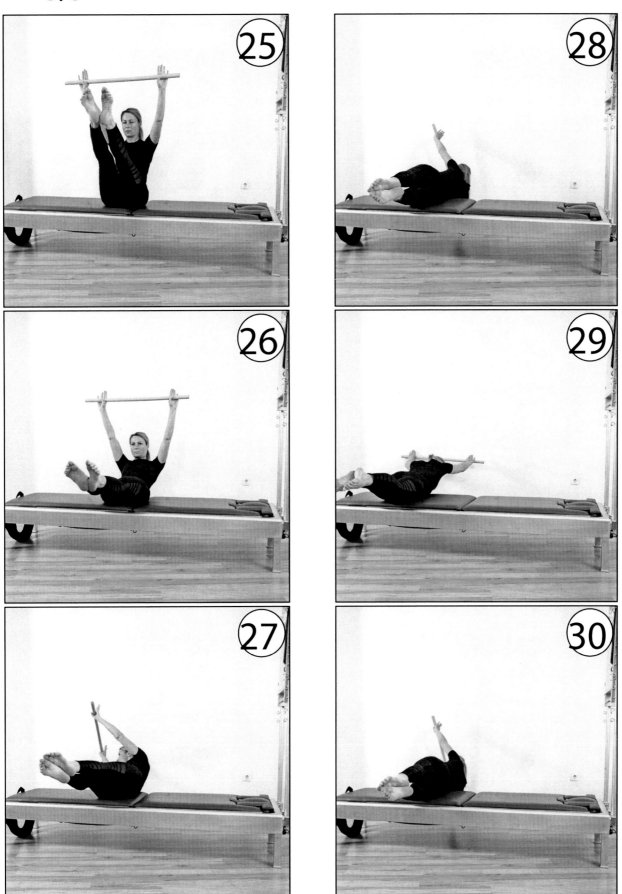

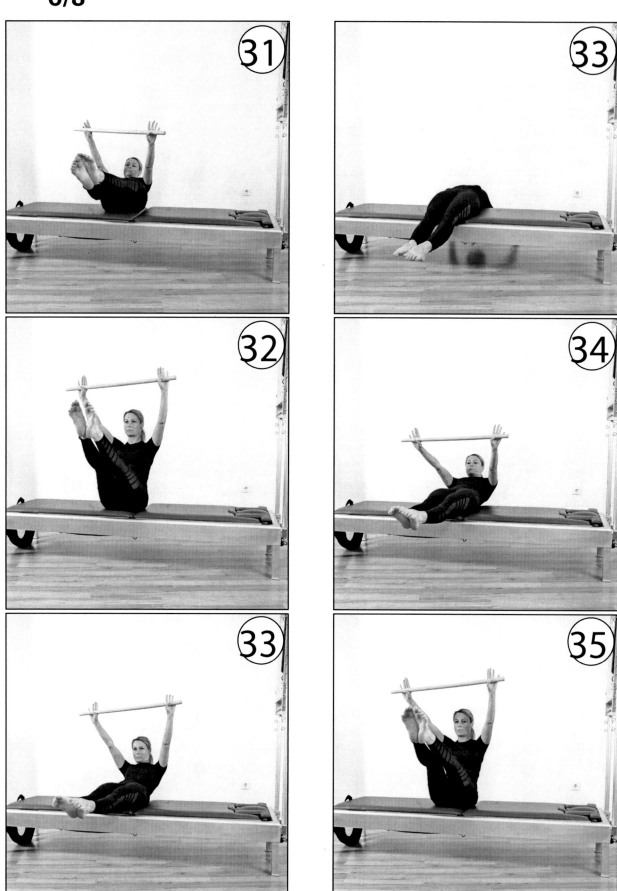

15. Teaser & Log Roll (T)
7/8

Setup:
Sit diagonally on the Cadillac mat with the knees bent and opened as far as necessary. The heels maintain the contact. The hands hold a bar in front of the shins. The palms face downward. Rounded lumbar spine. Choose a sitting position in which the tips of the shoulder blades are exactly on the edge of the Cadillac mat when rolled down completely.

Purpose of the Exercise:
Improvement of balance and coordination.
Strengthening of the hip flexors, entire abdominal musculature as well as the leg and back extensors.
Stretch of the abdominal muscles, shoulder muscles and hip flexors.
Opening of the thoracic and cervical spine.

Execution: 1x - 3x

Image 2-3: Come into the Teaser position, stretch the legs up to about 45 degrees and raise the arms with the bar until the arms are as close to the head as possible.

Image 4-6: Roll down slowly and in a controlled manner with the arms next to the ears and simultaneously lower the legs. Once the horizontal position has been reached, simultaneously lower the legs, the thoracic spine and the head into a controlled overextension. The arms are next to the head in the end position, if possible. Maintain inner abdominal tension.

Image 7-8: Come back the same way. Raise the arms and then the head and roll back up into the Teaser. Stretch the arms out to the front.

Image 9-11: Bend the legs and lift the feet over the bar (if possible simultaneously). In the Teaser, stretch the legs up to 45 degrees again. Place the bar below the thighs. Keep the arms stretched. If it is not possible to lift the feet over the bar, omit this exercise part including image 12 -14.

Image 12-14: Bend the legs and lift the feet (if possible simultaneously) over the bar. Stretch the legs up to approx. 45 degrees in the Teaser position and lift the arms with the bar so that the arms are as close to the head as possible.

Image 15-18: Roll down slowly and in a controlled manner with the arms next to the ears and simultaneously lower the legs. After reaching the horizontal, roll to the left in a controlled manner and from there into the prone position. Then, in the prone position, raise the legs, chest and arms.

Image 19-21: Roll back to the left side and from there into the Teaser again with the arms next to the ears.

Image 22-23: Bend the legs and lift the feet over the bar (if possible simultaneously). In the Teaser, stretch the legs up to 45 degrees again. Place the bar below the thighs. Keep the arms stretched. If it is not possible to lift the feet above the bar, omit this part of the exercise including image 24 -26.

Image 24-26: Bend the legs and lift the feet over the bar (if possible simultaneously). Stretch the legs up to approx. 45 degrees in the Teaser position and raise the arms with the bar so that the arms are as close to head as possible.

Image 27-29: Roll down slowly and in a controlled manner with the arms next to the ears and simultaneously lower the legs. After reaching the horizontal, roll to the right in a controlled manner and from there into the prone position. Then, in the prone position, raise the legs, chest and arms.

Image 30-32: Roll back onto the right side and from there back into the Teaser with the arms next to the ears.

Image 33-33: Roll down slowly and in a controlled manner with the arms next to the ears and simultaneously lower the legs. After reaching the horizontal, lower the legs, the thoracic spine and the head into a controlled overextension at the same time. The arms are next to the head in the end position, if possible. Maintain inner abdominal tension.

Image 34-35: Come back the same way. Raise the arms, then lift the head and finally roll back up into the Teaser. Stretch the arms out to the front.

15. Teaser & Log Roll (T)
8/8

Common Mistakes:

Image 6: Overstretching of the head and loss of control of the overextension through the abdominal muscles
Image 15-21 and 27 - 31: The Log Roll cannot be initiated from the inside. Preferably practice with the Cadillac Manual Part 1 Exercise "47. Roulade (M)" first.
Image 18 and 29: The raising of the legs, chest and arms is omitted.

Modifications or Variations:

At the end of the exercise, perform leg circles: Lower the legs, open them at the bottom, pull them apart and then bring them up into the starting position in a "D". Repeat 3x - 5x, then change the direction.

Contraindications/Risks:

Danger of falling off the Cadillac. If this danger exists during the exercise, try the exercise first without a bar on a High Mat or even on a Pilates mat on the floor.
Danger of a hollow back when raising the legs.

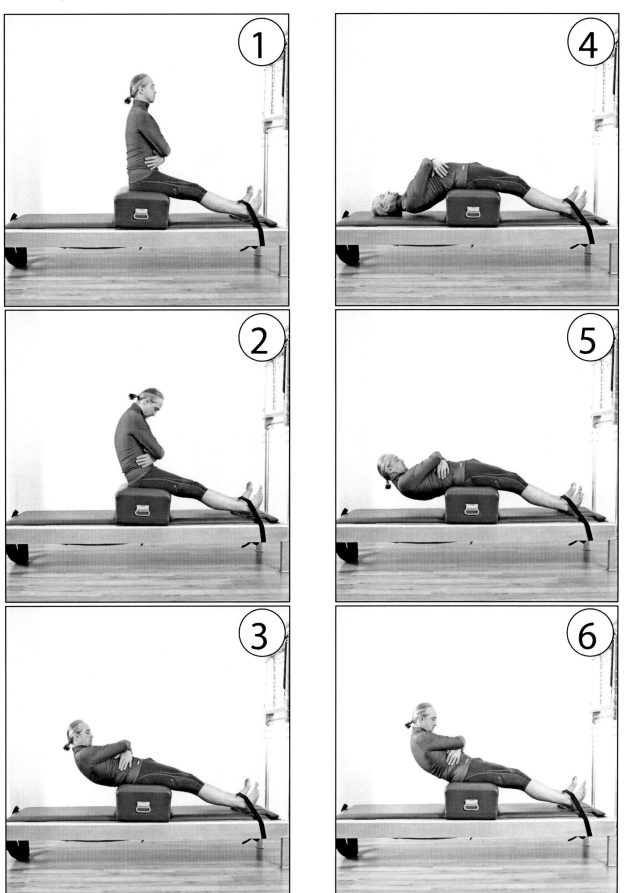

16. Short Box - Round (T)
2/3

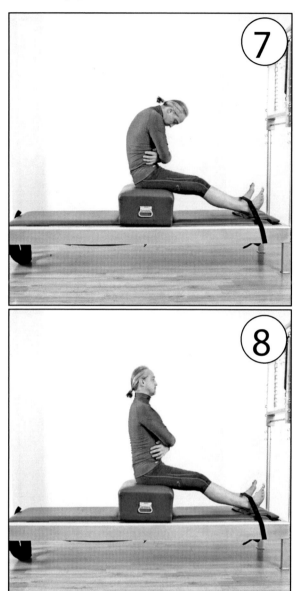

16. Short Box - Round (T)
3/3

Setup:
Place a Box diagonally on the Cadillac. When positioning the Box, make sure that the correct distance to the footstrap is chosen for the individual level of difficulty. Rule of thumb: The more stretched the legs are, the more demanding the exercise becomes.
Sitting on the Box so that one hand-width of space remains behind the buttocks. Stretch the feet below the footstrap, pull them to the sides and flex. Sit upright, gently bring the ischial tuberosities together, and pull out of the pelvis to reach maximum length. Place the left hand around the abdomen under the right ribs, and put the right hand on the left elbow.

Purpose of the Exercise:
Strengthening of the transversus abdominis, rectus abdominis and hip flexor.
Stretch of the hip flexor in the extension.
Mobilization of the spine.

Execution: 3x - 7x
Pull the abdomen inward, creating a large "C" curve with the shoulders above the hips. Then initiate the movement with a posterior pelvic tilt. Try to place the sacrum flat on the Box as early on as possible. Keep flexing the torso until the torso is parallel to the Cadillac mat. Gradually giving in, let the upper body sink down, maintaining a residual flexion in the cervical spine and thoracic spine. Gently place the head on the Cadillac mat.
Starting with the head, come back into the large "C" curve as early on during the roll-up as possible, and, maintaining it, come up until the shoulders are back above the hips. Only then sit upright again.

Common Mistakes:
Instead of lengthening the body and maintaining this length and the height (of the head) when getting into the "C" curve, the body curves in and becomes smaller.
After the horizontal has been reached, the head is overstretched to initiate the extension. It is better to keep the head in a flexion for as long as possible.
When rolling up, no "C" curve is reached and, instead, the upper body comes up in an extension or overextension of the lumbar spine. This usually indicates that the transversus abdominis is too weak and unable to sufficiently counteract the traction of the psoas at the lumbar spine.

Modifications or Variations:
Place the hands sideways next to the hip and grip the Box to support the pelvic tilt. Gradually loosen the grip and slide the hands over the Box.
Instead of working with the Box placed diagonally, place the Box horizontally. Nevertheless, sit at the front of the Box and, instead of using the strap, put the feet on the Cadillac mat. Only come down as far as you can also safely come back up without raising the legs.

Contraindications/Risks:
In case of a lack of abdominal stabilization, stop before reaching the horizontal and come back up. Risk of damaging the lumbar vertebrae.

17. Short Box - Flat (T)
1/2

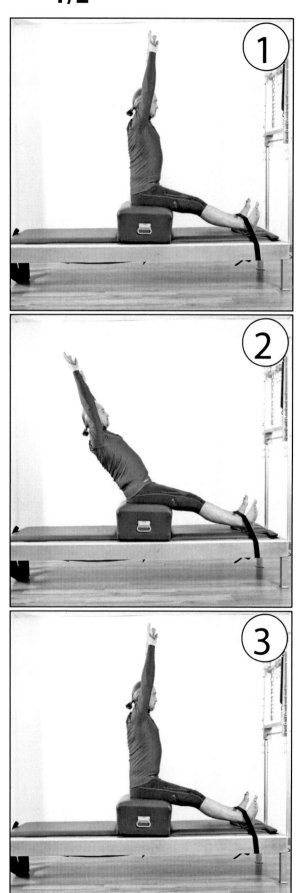

17. Short Box - Flat (T)
2/2

Setup:

Place a Box diagonally on the Cadillac. When positioning the Box, make sure that the correct distance to the footstrap is chosen for the individual level of difficulty. Rule of thumb: The more stretched the legs are, the more demanding the exercise becomes.

Sitting on the Box so that one hand width of space remains behind the buttocks. Stretch the feet below the footstrap, pull them to the sides and flex. The hands hold a bar slightly more than shoulder-wide apart and lightly pull away from each other. The arms are stretched upward. The exact height depends on the individual shoulder flexibility. Raise the arms only as far as no evasive movements are visible.

Sit upright, gently bring the ischial tuberosities together, and pull out of the pelvis to reach maximum length.

Purpose of the Exercise:

Strengthening of the entire abdominal musculature, back extensors, hip flexors, pelvic floor and shoulder.

Execution: 3x - 7x

Pull the abdomen inward. Initiate the movement with a posterior pelvic tilt and maintain the stability of the trunk. The pelvis and upper body form one unit. Lean back only as far as this stability can be properly maintained. The eyes keep looking at the opposite wall, but without bending the head forward. Then come back up. Try to stretch more and more, so that you feel bigger in the final position - with the shoulders above the hip - than before.

Common Mistakes:

Instead of lengthening the body and maintaining this length and the height (of the head) when getting into the "C" curve, the body curves in and becomes smaller.

The arms, holding the bar, are brought forward in relation to the torso to carry less weight. The head is pushed forward for the same reasons.

Coming back in a rounded position.

The eyes stop looking at the opposite wall.

Modifications or Variations:

Variations to make the exercise easier. Starting with the lightest version:
- Place the hands sideways next to the hip and grip the Box.
- The arms cross in front of the chest with the palms of the hands opened.
- The hands are clasped behind the head. Wide elbows.

A rolled towel, Thera-Band or Kathy Corey CORE Band® can also be used instead of the bar.

Instead of working with the Box placed diagonally, place the Box horizontally. Nevertheless, sit at the front of the Box and, instead of using the strap, put the feet on the Cadillac mat. Only come down as far as you can also safely come back up without raising the legs.

Contraindications/Risks:

Danger of a hollow back.

18. Short Box - Side-to-Side (T)
1/2

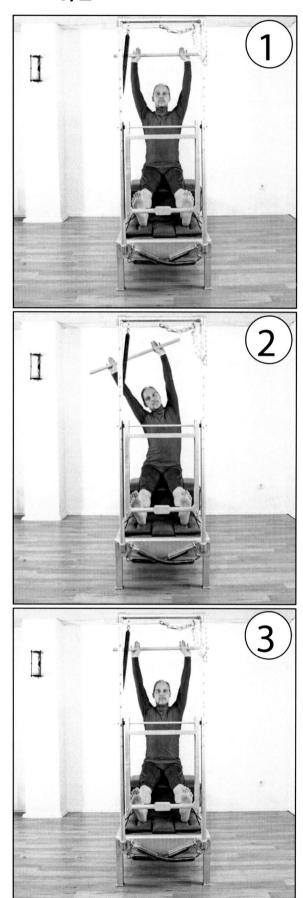

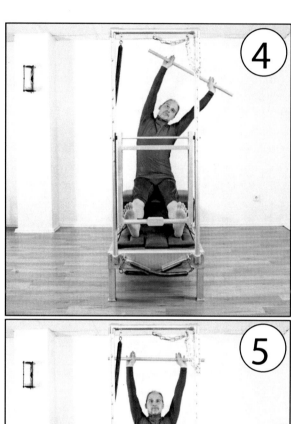

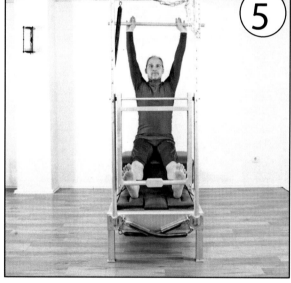

18. Short Box - Side-to-Side (T)
2/2

Setup:

Place a Box diagonally on the Cadillac. When positioning the Box, make sure that the correct distance to the footstrap is chosen for the individual level of difficulty. Rule of thumb: The more stretched the legs are, the more demanding the exercise becomes.

Sitting on the Box so that one hand width of space remains behind the buttocks. Stretch the feet below the footstrap, pull them to the sides and flex. The hands hold a bar slightly more than shoulder-wide apart and lightly pull away from each other. The arms are stretched upward. The exact height depends on the individual shoulder flexibility. Raise the arms only as far as no evasive movements are visible.

Sit upright, gently bring the ischial tuberosities together, and pull out of the pelvis to reach maximum length.

Purpose of the Exercise:

Stretch of the flank muscles (transversus abdominis, obliquus externus abdominis, obliquus internus abdominis, intercostalis, quadratus lomborum), back muscles, shoulders and intercostali.

Execution: 3x - 5x per side

Pull the abdomen inward. Bend to the right, as though bending over a large ball, and push the left side of the chest upward. Maintain equal weight on both buttocks. The arms keep the same distance to both ears. Stretch back into the center.

Bend to the left, as though bending over a large ball, and push the right side of the chest upward. Maintain equal weight on both buttocks. The arms keep the same distance to both ears. Stretch back into the center. The eyes keep looking at the opposite wall, but without bending the head forward.

Common Mistakes:

Instead of starting from the elongation, the body is not yet lengthened at the beginning of the movement.
During the lateral bending, the upper body is simultaneously rotated forward or backward.
The upper body leans back.
The arms come closer to the ear on the stretching side, since this feels like the body bends further.
The eyes stop looking at the opposite wall.
The ischial tuberosities lose contact with the Box.

Modifications or Variations:

The arms cross in front of the chest with the palms of the hands opened.
The hands are clasped behind the head. Wide elbows.
A rolled towel, Thera-Band or Kathy Corey CORE Band® can also be used instead of the bar.
Instead of working with the Box placed diagonally, place the Box horizontally. Nevertheless, sit at the front of the Box and, instead of using the strap, put the feet on the Cadillac mat. Only come down as far as you can also safely come back up without raising the legs.

Contraindications/Risks: -

19. Short Box - Twist prep (T)
1/2

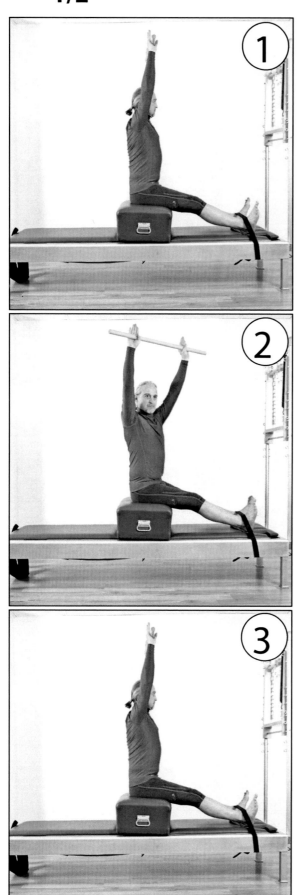

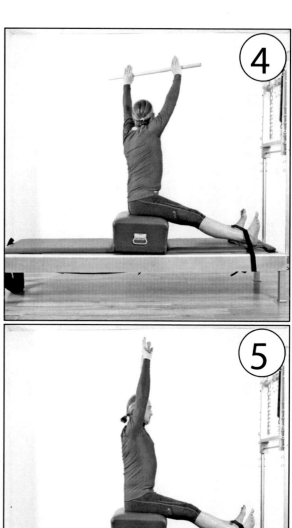

19. Short Box - Twist prep (T)
2/2

Setup:
Place a Box diagonally on the Cadillac. When positioning the Box, make sure that the correct distance to the footstrap is chosen for the individual level of difficulty. Rule of thumb: The more stretched the legs are, the more demanding the exercise becomes.

Sitting on the Box so that one hand width of space remains behind the buttocks. Stretch the feet below the footstrap, pull them to the sides and flex. The hands hold a bar slightly more than shoulder-wide apart and lightly pull away from each other. The arms are stretched upward. The exact height depends on the individual shoulder flexibility. Raise the arms only as far as no evasive movements are visible.

Sit upright, gently bring the ischial tuberosities together, and pull out of the pelvis to reach maximum length.

Purpose of the Exercise:
Alternately strengthening and stretching the Obliquus externus abdominis, Obliquus internus abdominis, pelvic floor, as well as the back muscles and shoulders.

Execution: 3x - 5x per side
Pull the abdomen inward. Turn to the right, feeling as though the lower left side of the ribs was initiating the movement. Lengthen the body. A sense of screwing upward. Support the movement with the exhalation. At the end of the movement, inhale to counter the cramping of the ribs. Maintaining the length, return to the center.

Turn to the left, with a feeling as though the lower right side of the ribs was initiating the movement. Lengthen the body. A sense of screwing upward. Support the movement with the exhalation. At the end of the movement, inhale to counter the cramping of the ribs. Maintaining the length, return to the center.

Common Mistakes:
Instead of starting from the elongation, the body is not yet lengthened at the beginning of the movement.
The upper body is simultaneously bent to one side during the rotation.
The upper body leans back.

Modifications or Variations:
The arms cross in front of the chest with the palms of the hands opened.
The hands are clasped behind the head. Wide elbows.
A rolled towel, Thera-Band or Kathy Corey CORE Band® can also be used instead of the bar.
Instead of working with the Box placed diagonally, place the Box horizontally. Nevertheless, sit at the front of the Box and, instead of using the strap, put the feet on the Cadillac mat.

Contraindications/Risks: -

20. Short Box - Twist & Reach (T)
1/3

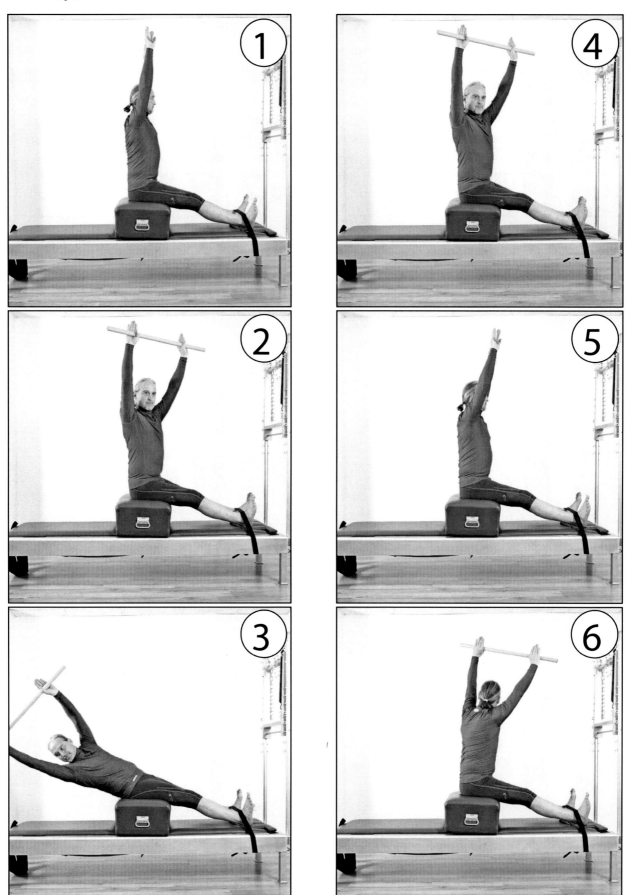

20. Short Box - Twist & Reach (T)
   2/3

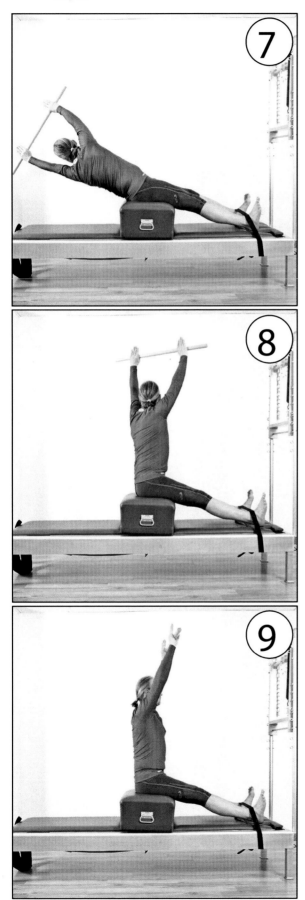

20. Short Box - Twist & Reach (T)
3/3

Setup:

Place a Box diagonally on the Cadillac. When positioning the Box, make sure that the correct distance to the footstrap is chosen for the individual level of difficulty. Rule of thumb: The more stretched the legs are, the more demanding the exercise becomes.

Sitting on the Box so that one hand width of space remains behind the buttocks. Stretch the feet below the footstrap, pull them to the sides and flex. The hands hold a bar slightly more than shoulder-wide apart and lightly pull away from each other. The arms are stretched upward. The exact height depends on the individual shoulder flexibility. Raise the arms only as far as no evasive movements are visible.

Sit upright, gently bring the ischial tuberosities together, and pull out of the pelvis to reach maximum length.

Purpose of the Exercise:

Strengthening of the hip flexors, Obliquus externus abdominis, Obliquus internus abdominis, back muscles, pelvic floor and shoulders.

Execution: 3x - 5x per side

Pull the abdomen inward. Turn to the right, feeling as though the lower left side of the ribs was initiating the movement. Lengthen the body. A sense of screwing upward. By tilting the pelvis into the direction of the right back edge of the Cadillac frame, lean backward. Come back up exactly the same way. Then rotate back to the center.

Turn to the left, feeling as though the lower right side of the ribs was initiating the movement. Lengthen the body. A sense of screwing upward. Maintaining the elongation, come back to the center. By tilting the pelvis into the direction of the left back edge of the Cadillac frame, lean backward. Come back up exactly the same way. Then rotate back to the center.

Common Mistakes:

Instead of starting from the elongation, the body is not yet lengthened at the beginning of the movement. The upper body is simultaneously bent to one side during the rotation.

While lowering laterally, the pelvic movement does not carry the movement out completely and, instead, a lateral bend with a hollow back occurs at a certain point.

The ischial tuberosities lose contact with the Box.

Modifications or Variations:

The arms cross in front of the chest with the palms of the hands opened.

The hands are clasped behind the head. Wide elbows.

A rolled towel, Thera-Band or Kathy Corey CORE Band® can also be used instead of the bar.

Magic Wand / Fishing Variation: At the end of the movement let go of the bar with the upper hand and use the lower hand to hold the bar as an extension of the upper body. Attention, there is a danger of hitting other people if the movement is performed in an uncontrolled manner.

From the horizontal, bend laterally without falling into the hollow back.

Instead of working with the Box placed diagonally, place the Box horizontally. Nevertheless, sit at the front of the Box, and, instead of using the strap, put the feet on the Cadillac mat.

Contraindications/Risks:

If the pelvis does not carry the movement out completely and a lateral bend with a hollow back occurs at a certain point instead, there can be muscle cramps in the back.

21. Short Box - Around the World (T)
   1/4

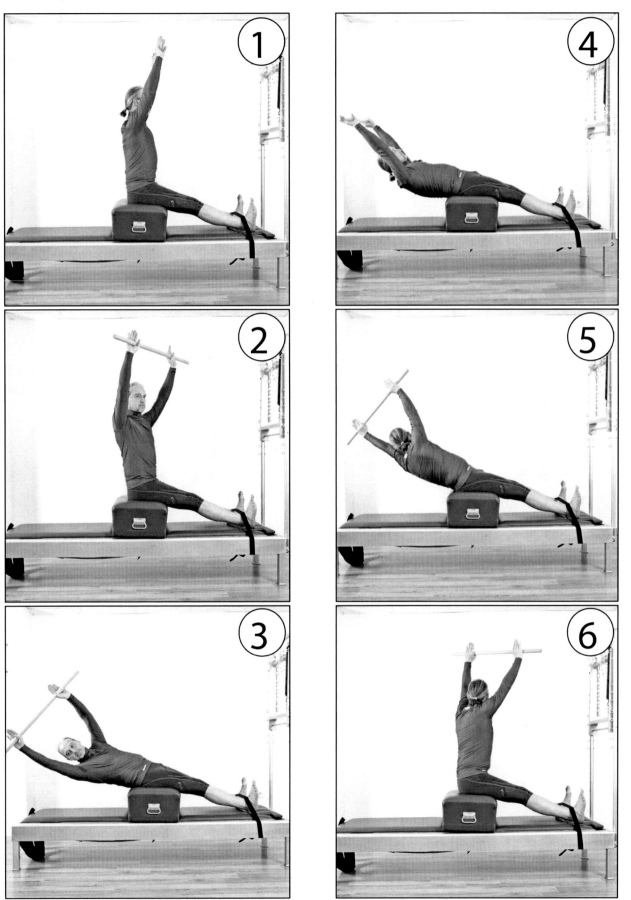

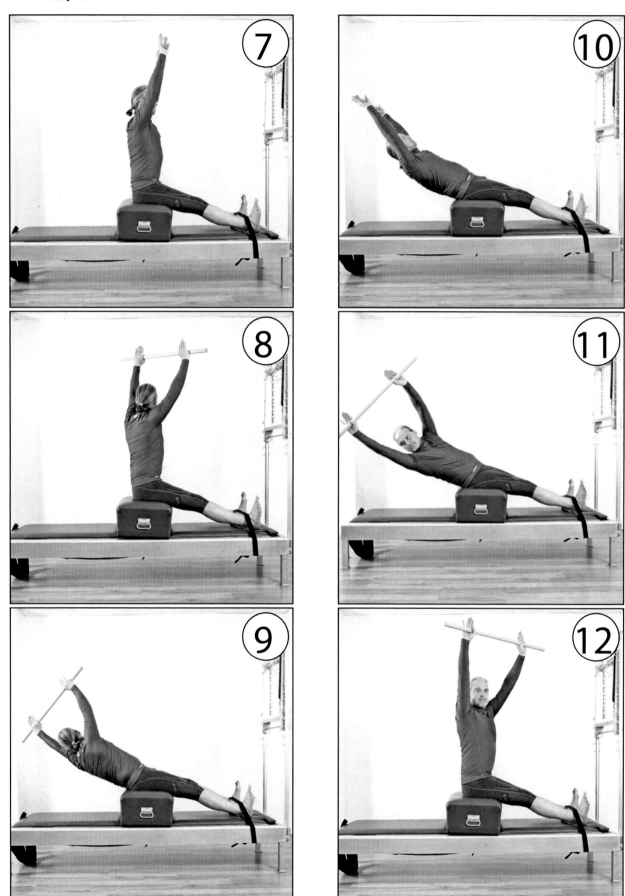

21. Short Box - Around the World (T)
3/4

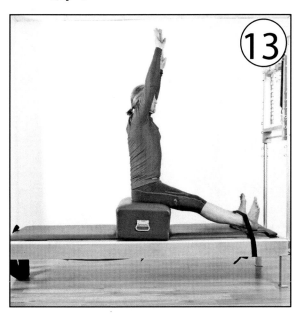

Setup:

Place a Box diagonally on the Cadillac. When positioning the Box, make sure that the correct distance to the footstrap is chosen for the individual level of difficulty. Rule of thumb: The more stretched the legs are, the more demanding the exercise becomes.

Sitting on the Box so that one hand width of space remains behind the buttocks. Stretch the feet below the footstrap, pull them to the sides and flex. The hands hold a bar slightly more than shoulder-wide apart and lightly pull away from each other. The arms are stretched upward. The exact height depends on the individual shoulder flexibility. Raise the arms only as far as no evasive movements are visible.

Sit upright, gently bring the ischial tuberosities together, and pull out of the pelvis to reach maximum length.

Purpose of the Exercise:

Strengthening of the hip flexors, back muscles, shoulders, external abdominal muscles, internal abdominal muscles and pelvic floor.

Execution: 3x - 5x per side

Pull the abdomen inward. Turn to the right, feeling as though the lower left side of the ribs was initiating the movement. Lengthen the body. A sense of screwing upward. By tilting the pelvis into the direction of the right back edge of the Cadillac frame, lean backward. In this position, rotate to the left side via the center. Come back up on the left side. Only when the body is fully upright again, turn back to the center.

Turn to the left, feeling as though the lower right side of the ribs was initiating the movement. Lengthen the body. A sense of screwing upward. By tilting the pelvis into the direction of the left back edge of the Cadillac frame, lean backward. In this position, rotate to the right side via the center. Come back up on the right side. Only when the body is fully upright again, turn back to the center.

21. Short Box - Around the World (T)
4/4

Common Mistakes:

Instead of starting from the elongation, the body is not yet lengthened at the beginning of the movement.
The upper body is simultaneously bent to one side during the rotation.
During the lateral lowering, the pelvis does not carry the movement out completely and, instead, a lateral bend with a hollow back occurs at a certain point.

Modifications or Variations:

The arms cross in front of the chest with the palms of the hands opened.
The hands are clasped behind the head. Wide elbows.
A rolled towel, Thera-Band or Kathy Corey CORE Band® can also be used instead of the bar.
From the horizontal, bend laterally without falling into the hollow back. In this position, rotate into an overextension via the center.
Instead of working with the Box placed diagonally, place the Box horizontally. Nevertheless, sit at the front of the Box and, instead of using the strap, put the feet on the Cadillac mat.
The ischial tuberosities lose their contact with the Box.

Contraindications/Risks:

If the pelvis does not carry the movement out completely and a lateral bend with a hollow back occurs at a certain point instead, then there can be muscle cramps in the back.

22. Short Box - Climb a Tree (T)
1/5

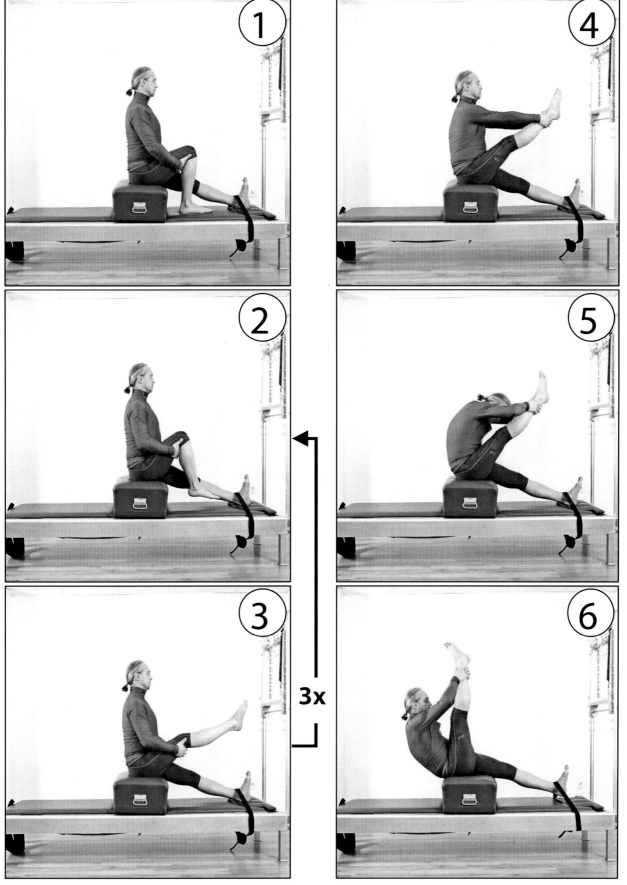

3x

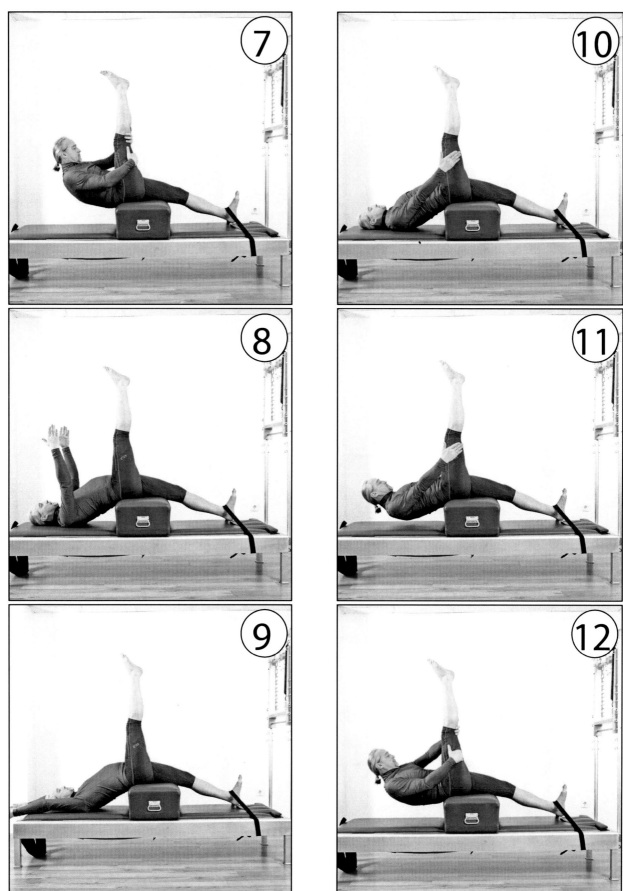

22. Short Box - Climb a Tree (T)
   3/5

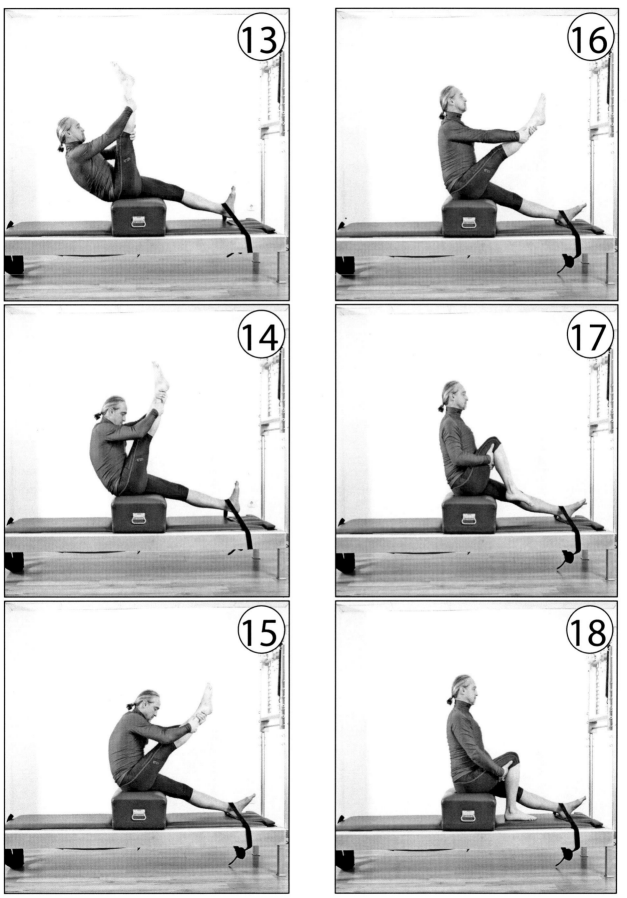

22. Short Box - Climb a Tree (T)
4/5

Setup:

Place a Box diagonally on the Cadillac. When positioning the Box, make sure that the correct distance to the footstrap is chosen for the individual level of difficulty. Rule of thumb: The more stretched the legs are, the more demanding the exercise becomes.

Sitting on the Box so that one hand width of space remains behind the buttocks. Stretch the feet below the footstrap, pull them to the sides and flex. The hands hold a bar slightly more than shoulder-wide apart and lightly pull away from each other. The arms are stretched upward. The exact height depends on the individual shoulder flexibility. Raise the arms only as far as no evasive movements are visible.

Sit upright, gently bring the ischial tuberosities together, and pull out of the pelvis to reach maximum length.

Purpose of the Exercise:

Strengthening of the transversus abdominis, rectus abdominis and the hip flexor.
Stretch of the leg backside, which is being moved.
Stretch of the hip flexor with the foot in the strap in the extension.

Execution: 1- 3x per side

Place the right foot closely in front of the Box, the left foot remains below the strap. With both hands, grip below the right thigh, closely to the knees. Maintain the upright position of the spine. Now pull the right knee toward the chest as far as possible without sinking in with the lumbar spine or leaning backward.

Loosely stretch the right leg three times. Maintaining the back extension and the thigh height is more important than stretching the leg completely. This part of the exercise is a slight pre-stretch. During the third stretch repetition, keep the right leg stretched and climb up the leg with the hands in three "steps", coming as close as possible to the ankle. Round the back and pull the head down toward the leg without simultaneously lowering the leg. At the same time pull the abdomen away from the right thigh.

While maintaining this position, lean back by tilting the pelvis until the right leg is vertical. Climb down the leg in three steps. Now, the hands let go of the leg and the upper body gradually sinks downward, maintaining a residual flexion in the cervical and thoracic spine. Gently place the head on the Cadillac mat. Move the arms backward and then forward again in a circular arc, toward the right leg.

Roll up, starting with the head. When the upper body is horizontal, grip the right leg with the hands and climb up to the ankle in three "steps" again. Now, holding the position, come up until the shoulders are above the hips. Try to straighten up the upper body as much as possible. Then, in three "steps", climb down the leg and bring the hands to the hollow of the knee again. For only one repetition, put the right foot down onto the mat again. For two more repetitions, start again directly with the three-fold stretching of the leg. After 3 repetitions, switch sides.

Common Mistakes:

Instead of lengthening the body and maintaining this length and the height (of the head) when getting into the "C" curve, the body curves in and becomes smaller.

The back gives in and rounds when the right leg is raised/extended for the first time.

After the horizontal has been reached, the head is overstretched to initiate the extension. It is better to keep the head in a flexion for as long as possible.

The head hangs down while rolling up.

22. Short Box - Climb a Tree (T)
5/5

Modifications or Variations:

When the shoulder is above the hip again in image 15, pull the right foot above the head: "Cherry picking". Instead of working with the Box placed diagonally, place the Box horizontally. Nevertheless, sit at the front of the Box and, instead of using the strap, put the feet on the Cadillac mat.

Contraindications/Risks:

After letting go of the leg with the hands, considerable pressure can be exerted on the lumbar spine. This should only be done with healthy and sufficient preliminary Pilates training.

Acknowledgments

First of all I would like to thank my wife and my children, who had to see their husband and father sit behind the laptop for many days, while this second part was being created. From the first photo shooting to the second part, which is now available, more than 2 years have passed. In this time my daughter changed from the role of the observer to the editor of this book and translator of the first and now second part of the manual. A special thank you for her tireless efforts.

A further, special thank you to my parents, who have always supported my various changes in sports and theories of movement, and who did not bat an eyelid when I opened a Shaolin Weng Chun Kung Fu School first thing after completing my psychology studies. I dedicate this second part of the training manual to them.

I would also like to thank my first Pilates teacher, Mario Alfonso, and my Pilates instructor, Miriam Friedrich Honorio, whose deep understanding of movement and especially of the quality of movement influenced me significantly. I also thank Alexandra Clasen, whose Gyrotonic Studio is my refuge week after week. With her I can break down the topic of movement from a different perspective than Pilates.

I particularly want to thank Kathy Corey, who has greatly expanded my knowledge about the possibilities of the Cadillac during my 2-year mentoring program with her.

Further special thanks go to Alice Talkington, who has taken it upon herself to review all the traditional exercises of the manual with regard to the correct naming.

I would further like to thank my two co-authors: Dr. Ingo Barck and Felicitas Ruthe. Without the many hours of work they put into this manual and their irreplaceable input, the manual would have been impossible to complete in such a detailed way.

Many thanks also to my wonderful photo models Helena Klimtova, Frank Staude and Claudia Holtmanns, who exercised and sweated with us for hours to provide the necessary pictures for the manual. Their radiant smiles and stamina not only enriched this manual but truly made it possible in the first place.

Finally, I want to thank my clients, apprentices and teachers at pilates-powers. Without the possibility of exploring, deconstructing and rediscovering all of the Pilates exercises with different types of bodies every single day, this manual would not exist.

Thank you!

Toenisvorst, October 2019   Reiner Grootenhuis

About the Author

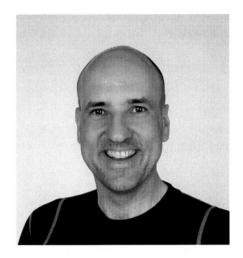

Besides obtaining a diploma in psychology, Reiner Grootenhuis has studied the healing and martial arts of the Southern Shaolin Monastery - Weng Chun.

After completing his psychology studies in 1992, he founded a Weng Chun Kung Fu School in Wuerzburg and ran it until 1995. After selling his martial arts school, he continued to teach self-defense to women and children.

Due to his work as an executive, as well as his part-time MBA studies and lecturing, Kung Fu and other sports activities increasingly disappeared into the background.

Reiner was looking for an alternative, holistic system to get fit again and found what he was looking for with Pilates in 2005. Parallel to his professional activities, he completed his training as a Pilates trainer for mats and equipment at the Pilates training institute BASI (Body Arts & Science International).

He is the founder and manager of the world's largest Pilates forum, pilates-contrology-forum on Facebook, with over 10,00 Pilates teachers worldwide.

In March 2012 he opened the pilates-powers studio in Toenisvorst, near Dusseldorf.

In June 2014 Reiner participated in the Master Mentor Program with BASI founder Rael Isacowitz.

At the end of 2014 he was appointed to the Board of Directors of the Pilates Heritage Congress by Kathy Corey. The congress takes place every 2 years in the birthplace of Joseph Pilates, Moenchengladbach.

Since 2014 he has been offering his own Pilates training program, the graduates and students of which have already opened their own studios.

In July 2017, Reiner completed Kathy Corey's two-year Master Mentor Program and has been awarded the title of a "Kathy Corey Pilates Master Teacher" in July 2019

Since November 2017 Reiner is also a Pilates Intel Expert for the online magazine Pilates Intel for which he regularly writes articles.

In September 2018 Reiner has been nominated as a member of the Certification Committee of the German Pilates Association.

In 2015 he published the first publicly accessible German training manual for the Wunda Chair and in 2016 the first training manual in the world about the Arm Chair inspired by MeJo Wiggin. In 2018, part one of the Cadillac Manual was published in German, and 2019 in English.

About the Co-Authors

Biography Dr. Ingo Barck

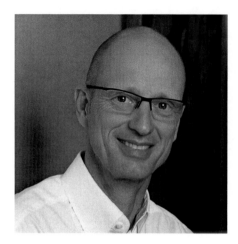

Dr. Ingo Barck has always been a passionate athlete. Throughout his life, he has performed various sports such as swimming, athletics, rowing, handball, underwater rugby, diving, paragliding, kite surfing, triathlon, and judo (certified instructor/long-standing work as a trainer). Today he enjoys running, swimming, bicycle racing, inline skating, skiing, wakeboarding and, since 2013, Pilates.

The certified medical doctor was able to gain experience in orthopedics and surgery, as well as some insight into the industry in 2007, before he started working as a manual therapist for pain patients in his own private medical practice. He particularly focuses on the connective tissue (fasciae), which has gained increasing recognition over the past few years.

Biography Felicitas Ruthe

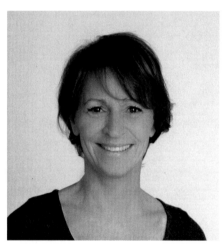

Felicitas is a certified occupational therapist and, as part of her work, has completed a Bobath training and further education in the areas of Affolter (treatment of children with perceptual disorders through manual guidance), basal stimulation, Feldenkrais and back training.

Felicitas came to Pilates in 2012 through her husband, with whom she participated in a Pilates course at pilates-powers. Due to her own positive experiences, she decided to start her Pilates education at pilates-powers in March 2014, which she successfully completed in April 2017. Her thesis deals with the pelvic floor, its problems, and how Pilates can make an impact. In her lessons, she combines her functional knowledge from occupational therapy with the Pilates method.

About the Photo Models

Biography Helena Klimtova

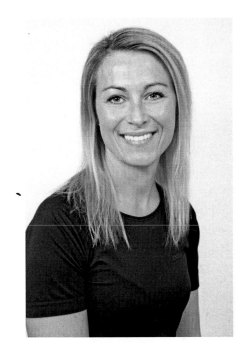

Helena came to Pilates at the beginning of 2015, and it convinced her so much that she decided to study Pilates at the pilates-powers studio.

"Pilates brought me back my agility and flexibility, which I had acquired through 12 years of gymnastics and rhythmic gymnastics, but lost again through work and the birth of my two children. During Pilates, I feel that I truly have my body under control. I feel much safer, even during other sports, such as skiing or running. What I love about Pilates are the many possibilities, the different equipment, and the many exercises, especially the numerous variations of the exercises (thank you, Reiner).

I look forward to my training every day because I know that I can achieve even more with Pilates. Pilates truly is my "happy hour", and I want to share it with my customers in my 'Fit Pilates' studio in Kaldenkirchen."

Biography Frank Staude

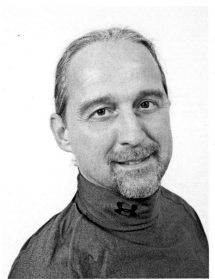

Frank Staude had been doing sports since his youth, starting with artistic and then trampoline gymnastics with national and international success. After his active time on the national team, he tried many sports to keep my body flexible and fit.

"I rather coincidentally discovered Pilates almost five years ago and had my first try-out lesson. I have been thrilled ever since to have finally found the sport in which I can combine everything I have been looking for: To train strength, stretching, stability and control in small groups with the attention of well-educated instructors, as well as having a lot of variety through the use of different exercises on equipment without weights. Today, I determine and control what is possible. Over and over again I am surprised to see how much mobility can be regained."

About the Photo Models (continued)

Biography Claudia Holtmanns

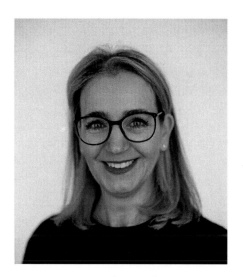

Claudia Holtmanns, born in 1967, tried various sports as a child. In the end she stuck with gymnastics. After she made it to the city champion in this sport in the highest compulsory class, she decided to give up on competitive sport, founded a dance club at her school and completed her training as an aerobics trainer in 1986. Over the next 10 years she saw many trends come and go.

When she first read a report about Pilates in Vogue in the late 90s, she initially suspected only another trend from America. But the more she learned about it, the more she was fascinated by the method. She first trained with Pilates Coach, Juliana Afram and Polestar. But the more she learned, the more certain she became that there was so much more behind it.

So, in 2009, she contacted Lolita San Miguel, who had developed a Master Mentor Program, and asked if Mrs San Miguel could offer this program in Germany as well. Since Claudia lives only a few kilometers away from Joseph Pilates' birthplace, Moenchengladbach, Lolita agreed. Claudia brought together 12 participants for the PMMP in 4 months and rented the Kaiser Friedrich Hall in Moenchengladbach for 2 hours on the first Saturday in May to celebrate the Pilates Day there together with almost 100 participants from all over Germany - these were the conditions of Mrs San Miguel. This event was the birth of the Pilates Heritage Congress, which brought together participants from 43 nations in Moenchengladbach in 2019.

Through the close cooperation with Lolita, she got to know Kathy Corey in 2011. Fascinated by the range and depth of her experience, it was clear to her that she also wanted to participate in the Post Graduate Program with Kathy. Hence, she traveled to Switzerland with Reiner for the first time in January 2016, and both agreed after the first day that they could still learn an incredible amount from Kathy, who had worked with all the Elders. This collaboration continues to this day, even though the program already ended in 2017.

Claudia has had her studio in Meerbusch for almost 15 years and now offers Pilates in individual and group training in 3 training rooms on almost 300 square meters.

She developed her own training program and will become a teacher educator for Kathy Corey's Basic Program starting in 2020.

Claudia is married, has 4 adult children with her husband and lives in Krefeld with her family (and dog).

Photo Shoot Locations

Find Yourself GmbH, Meerbusch

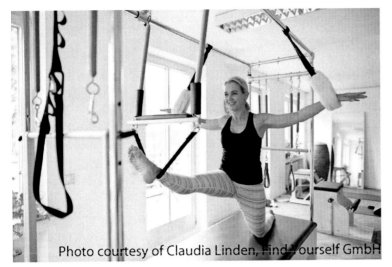

Photo courtesy of Claudia Linden, Find Yourself GmbH

The studio is located in Meerbusch near Düsseldorf . What started as a sublet in a ballet studio, developed over the years - and after moving twice - into a spacious studio with almost 300 square meters of training space in 3 classrooms fully equipped with Balanced Body equipment. The studio closed at the end of July 2020 after more than 15 years for personal reasons.

The owner, Claudia Linden (formerly Holtmanns), has completed the PMMP of Lolita San Miguel and further participated in the Post Graduate Education Program of Kathy Corey, which she hosts in Meerbusch herself. She is also a board member of the International Heritage Conference, which takes place in Moenchengladbach every two years.

pilates-powers, Toenisvorst

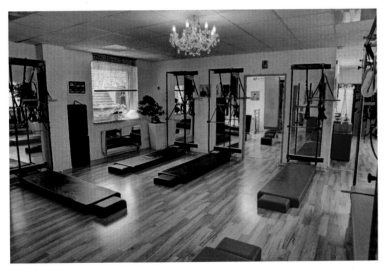

Founded in 2012 by Reiner Grootenhuis, the studio quickly became an insider tip for both customers and Pilates trainers in the area. With 46 hours of Pilates lessons a week and training certified according to the strict criteria of the German Pilates Association, it is a small Pilates paradise.

All Pilates equipment created by Joseph Pilates can be found at pilates-powers. Besides, one can try Pilates equipment from different manufacturers. This allows you to perform the same exercise using different equipment and to quickly discover the advantages and disadvantages of each manufacturer. In addition, pilates-powers probably has one of the most extensive Pilates libraries of all. The rooms, which are located in an old coffin factory, have a high degree of cosiness, which is highly appreciated by customers and trainers.